*WORKING WITH EMOTIONS
IN PSYCHOTHERAPY*

THE PRACTICING PROFESSIONAL
A Guilford Series
Edited by
MICHAEL J. MAHONEY

SELF-NARRATIVES: THE CONSTRUCTION OF MEANING
IN PSYCHOTHERAPY
Herbert J. M. Hermans and Els Hermans-Jansen

FOCUSING-ORIENTED PSYCHOTHERAPY: A MANUAL
OF THE EXPERIENTIAL METHOD
Eugene T. Gendlin

WORKING WITH DREAMS IN PSYCHOTHERAPY
Clara E. Hill

WORKING WITH EMOTIONS IN PSYCHOTHERAPY
Leslie S. Greenberg and Sandra C. Paivio

Working with Emotions in Psychotherapy

LESLIE S. GREENBERG
and
SANDRA C. PAIVIO

THE GUILFORD PRESS
New York   London

©1997 The Guilford Press
A Division of Guilford Publications, Inc.
72 Spring Street, New York, NY 10012

Printed in the United States of America

This book is printed on acid-free paper.

Last digit is print number: 9 8 7 6 5 4 3 2 1

Library of Congress Cataloging-in-Publication Data

Greenberg, Leslie S.
  Working with emotions in psychotherapy / Leslie S.
Greenberg
      p.   cm. — (The Practicing Professional)
  Includes bibliographical references and index.
  ISBN 1-57230-243-7
  1. Emotions. 2. Psychotherapy 3. Personal construct
theory. I. Paivio, Sandra C. II. Title. III. Series.
RC489.E45G74   1997
616.89′14—dc21   97–13521
                                                             CIP

To Brenda, Ari, and Teya (L. G.),
and Jerry, Maija-lisa, and Katlin (S. P.),
who have given us a lot of love,
joy, excitement, anger, sadness, fear,
and no shame. You have taught us
a lot about our own emotions.

Preface

WE ARE ENTERING a new era—the era of the scientifically based study of emotion. Once one has seen a PET scan that shows different areas of the brain lighting up for different emotions, or one area becoming active when a person is having flashbacks, and another added when these become more regulated memories, there is no going back. Emotion is an empirical fact, both experientially and scientifically.

Emotions move us and inform us, and when they are integrated with reason, they make us wiser than we are when we use our intellects alone. Although a lot has been written about cognition and reason in psychotherapy, not that much has been said about emotion. This book begins to restore the balance. In so doing, it gives reason and reflection their appropriate role in human change processes and experience. Ideally, reason and reflection guide emotion and work in the service of affective goals to resolve problems related to well-being.

We hope in the future to see many more books based on the empirical observation of different emotions in the treatment of psychological disorders. This book is just the beginning of the investigation of emotion in psychotherapy. We have chosen to focus on those emotions that are frequently observed in individual therapies—namely, the unpleasant emotions of anger, sadness, fear, and shame, and the more pleasant ones of joy, interest/excitement, and love (the emotion no one understands, but all wish to experience). We look forward to studies of psychotherapeutic work with rage, envy, jealousy, contempt, guilt, remorse, pride, and hope in individual, couple, and family therapy. We also look forward to studies of emotions in different problem contexts, such as depression, anxiety, childhood maltreatment, couple conflict, parenting, and so on.

One of the great puzzles about psychotherapy is that many different approaches work for many different people and for many different problems. This has led to the exploration of psychotherapy integration. We offer this book in the spirit of integration. In the formation of an applied human science, it will be important to understand the roles of emotion, motivation, cognition, behavior, and their interaction, as well as those of biochemistry and social systems.

The therapeutic relationship and the working alliance between therapist and client already have been shown to be key factors in therapeutic effectiveness. These constitute true common factors that cut across approaches. We offer emotional processes as additional important factors to be considered in the integration of therapeutic endeavors. First, the emotional bond is central in the formation of a therapeutic relationship and alliance. In addition, emotion is the basis of both experience and personal meaning. In working with people's past and present personal meaning and experience, and in providing them with new experience and new personal meaning, all therapies work with emotions. Working with emotions is thus central to psychotherapy.

We have provided tables in Chapters 3 and 6 that summarize the essential elements of our approach to assessment of emotional states and the framework for intervention. This is the best way to quickly get to the heart of our integrative approach to working with emotions. Reading Chapters 1, 3, and 6 will provide the necessary background for understanding these tables. A more detailed description of the book and of the contents of each chapter is given at the end of Chapter 1.

We would like to thank Kitty Moore, who helped us shape a volume twice the size of the present one into a more readable form, and Mike Mahoney for his continued support and feedback. We also thank our untiring secretary, Zehra Bandhu, for typing yet another seemingly endless manuscript. Next, we offer our heartfelt thanks to all of the students (some of whom are already valued colleagues) who have contributed to our thinking and practice. Many of them were therapists in our studies. Those with whom we currently are connected include Kristen Adams, Liz Bolger, Jonathan Carryer, Tom Chapeskie, Florence Foerster, Shari Geller, Rhonda Goldman, Karen Hirscheimer, Lorne Korman, Wanda Malcolm, Shelly McMain, Jim Nieuwenhuis, Lorraine Patterson, Rebecca Pederson, Kevin Rice, Ruth Rohn, Lana Shimp, Malinhi Singh, Serine Warwar, Janis Weston, and Bill Whelton. We also thank the following colleagues for continued support and shared commitment to studying the therapeutic process: Lynne Angus, Robert Elliott, Sue Johnson, Juan Pascual-Leone, Dave Rennie, Shake' Toukmanian, and Jeanne Watson. Finally, we extend our warmest thanks to all our clients.

Contents

Contents

WORKING WITH EMOTIONS
IN PSYCHOTHERAPY

CHAPTER ONE

The Centrality of Emotion in Psychotherapy

*T*HIS BOOK EXPLORES the role of emotion in psychotherapeutic change. The view that emotional arousal is an important common factor in psychotherapy was initially expressed by Frank (1963) in his seminal thinking on persuasion and healing. Since then, it has become clear to many experienced therapists and psychological theorists alike that the affective system is critical, both in understanding and in changing human experience and behavior.

One of our goals in this book is to promote the integration of the treatment of emotion, motivation, cognition, and behavior into a comprehensive approach to treatment (Norcross & Goldfried, 1992). Indeed, emotion awareness and its arousal and reorganization have been increasingly recognized as critical to psychotherapeutic change in many therapeutic approaches. Thus promoting emotional processing in cognitive approaches, arousal of fear by imaginal stimulation in behavioral approaches, emotional insight in psychodynamic approaches, increased depth of experiencing in experiential approaches, and communication of feelings in interactional approaches are all aspects of working with emotion that are seen as important within each perspective.

In this book we will show how therapists can think about and intervene with emotion in differential ways. First, they need to recognize the relationship between emotion and cognition. Emotion is intimately connected with meaning, and no emotional change takes place without producing cognitive change. This view informs the therapeutic process in clear ways. Second, therapists need to recognize

1

that emotional experience and expression can stem from different states of mind. For example, sadness due to the loss of a loved one differs from sadness due to violation or trauma. Therapeutic intervention will correspondingly differ. Third, the expression of certain emotions such as rage often stems from a more fundamental experience such as shame. Thus the client furious at his wife may be harboring another layer of feelings that the therapist needs to access.

Finally, each emotion—sadness, anger, and so forth—has its own characteristics, and there are different ways of working with each. Newly acknowledged anger and sadness, for example, often provide healthy adaptive information. The overly pleasing client who is able to access anger becomes more assertive and is able to stand up for her- or himself. Fear and shame, however, generally inhibit and are accessed in therapy not for their adaptive information but in order to make them more accessible to new experience and change. Clients who have suffered abuse and who revisit their fear and shame with the protection of the therapist can access present resources that help them to transform these feelings. Other emotions such as explosive anger and punitive self-contempt in turn need to be regulated often by self-soothing. Pleasant emotions, such as interest/excitement, joy, and love, are often end products of the process of resolving other emotional states. Appreciation, for example, often can only arise after resentment has been expressed and acknowledged. The pleasant emotions also act as antidotes to the unpleasant emotions. Thus each emotion is worked with in different ways.

The essence of our approach to treatment involves the establishment of an emotionally focused empathic dialogue between two people in which the therapist is attuned to, stimulates, and focuses on the clients' emotional concerns. In working with clients' emotion it is both the empathic, validating, relationship and the continual focus on accessing and reorganizing of emotional experience that are the core ingredients of effective psychotherapy.

This book presents a three-phase framework for working with emotion. This framework was devised by analyzing the tapes of a large number of successful emotionally focused therapies of depressed and anxious clients, as well as clients with interpersonal problems and general problems in living (Paivio & Greenberg, 1995; Greenberg & Watson, in press). We studied the tapes to ascertain how these clients actually changed and what therapists did to facilitate this process (Greenberg & Foerster, 1996; Watson & Greenberg, 1996). We identified three phases—bonding, evoking and exploring emotional experience, and emotion restructuring—each involving a number of specific steps designed to achieve the aim of that phase.

EMOTION SCHEMES

In our model of functioning the basic psychological unit or generating mechanism of emotional experience and meaning is what we call the "emotion scheme."[1] A scheme involves a set of organizing principles, constructed from the individual's innate response repertoire and past experience, that interact with the current situation and generate current experience. Schemes are highly personal and idiosyncratic, laden with emotional memories, hopes, expectations, fears, and knowledge gleaned from lived experience. We therefore call them personal or emotion schemes. Not based solely on emotion, they involve a complex synthesis of affect, cognition, motivation, and action that provides each person with an integrated sense of him- or herself and the world, as well as with subjective felt meaning (Greenberg & Safran, 1987; Greenberg, Rice, & Elliott, 1993).

These emotion schemes profoundly influence experience, behavior, and interaction. People have different emotional schemes associated with relationships with significant individuals in their lives. For example, being with one's mother may evoke a scheme of being anxious, or playful, or of feeling dread. Likewise, people can have different schemes attached to performing a task, such as feeling inept, effective, or undermined. Obviously, there are an infinite number of unique emotional schemes.

As therapists, we wish to stay as close as possible to the client's scheme generated subjective experience. This experience differs from the more logical rationality of reality representations. Personal experience is characterized by being affectively charged, and is obviously not an identical representation of events in external reality. Indeed, our schemes are not internalized replicas of the external world, but rather they are models constructed out of our own experience and action of being in the world. Moreover, a significant amount of coding of experience exists at the nonverbal level, and it is more concerned with being and doing than with conscious conceptual knowing. Emotional memory is thus laden with perceptual, sensory, and kinaesthetic aspects. Our first childhood memories, for example, are filled with feelings, sensations, sights, sound, and smells far more than with verbalized beliefs. A personal or emotion scheme thus is a record of subjective lived experience. It serves both as a basic format for remembering affective experience and for integrating the whole experience into a meaningful unity.

---

[1]We use the word "scheme" rather than "schema" to emphasize the action-oriented, rather than representational, nature of a scheme (Greenberg et al., 1993).

Our basic contention is that personal reality and consciousness is as much a product of emotions as it is of thought and rationality. In our view automatic emotion responses often precede or influence the conscious meanings of events. It is the high-level emotional meaning of events, constructed automatically by emotion schemes, that determines both conscious emotional and cognitive responses. This high-level "sense" of things is deeply affective in nature. It is the emotion scheme's function to read affectively relevant patterns from the environment and to guide both our emotional sense of ourselves and our orientation to the world. This guiding self-structure is only amenable to change once it has been activated. It is then that we experience our emotions, and the associated cognitions are "hot."

EMOTIONS IN THERAPY

A crucial aspect of development, and of therapy, is to promote the integration of people's basic affective experience and emotion into their existing organizations of their experience. The integration in therapy of basic affect into our self-organization involves tasks of differentiating, symbolizing, owning, and articulating our bodily felt emotional experience, allowing and accepting our emotions, learning to use our emotions as signals, and being able to synthesize different and contradictory emotions in response to the same person or situation. Engaging in these tasks is often aided by another's empathic attunement to our feelings. Integrating our emotional experience into existing personal structures leads to a stronger more integrated sense of self.

Emotions provide a rich source of information about our reactions to situations. Emotions, or more accurately those constituents of emotions that may have been out of awareness, can be brought into awareness to enhance the way in which we evaluate our needs, desires, goals, and concerns. What is required, particularly in therapy, is an understanding of what emotions indicate to us about the way in which we are conducting our lives.

We will suggest that it is only through accessing emotion and emotional meaning that emotional problems can be cured and that purely rational methods, although sometimes useful, too often do not cure distressed emotion. Reason has never succeeded in controlling passion. Moral imperatives or reasoned argument only succeed in regulating emotion when they themselves become emotional. Given that it is high-level emotion schemes that produce personal meaning, we will argue that it is these tacit emotion schemes that need to be accessed and changed to create new meaning. Merely expressing emotion however will often not correct situations. Rather, one needs to read the message of one's own emotional experience and use it as a guide to constructive action.

In therapy certain types of emotions are seen as curative in themselves. Primary emotional responses are creatively organizing because they help set new goal priorities. Thus when we help clients to attend to and symbolize their primary experience—their sadness, anger, or joy—this helps them access important needs/goals/concerns and helps them create new meaning. For example, once a client recognizes the hurt underlying his anger and thrust for dominance, he begins to be able to seek the comfort he really needs. When a man who suffers panic attacks recognizes his momentary fear of being abandoned as the trigger of his phobic chain of experience, he begins to find new ways of dealing with his fears of abandonment. When a woman acknowledges her anger at being shamed, she begins to mobilize assertively in protection of her self. Although emotions organize us for action and build up new adaptive structures, they are also involved in the breaking down of old static structures. Thus at times we need to evoke traumatic emotional memories in order to reprocess and restructure them. In addition, old emotional habits such as rage following shame, and fear following intimacy, have to be activated in therapy in order to be reorganized. For clients with underregulated shame or anger, symbolization of emotion helps transform these emotions. Symbolizing feelings and emotions provides a safe distance that prevents the person from feeling overwhelmed or acting out and sets the stage for learning how to soothe the fragile self.

In addition, therapy involves developing adaptive emotion-regulation strategies. This is done in therapy by repeating developmental sequences similar to the ones of a healthy childhood. Clients in therapy learn to self-regulate their emotions through the internalization of soothing interactions with the therapist and developing self-empathy. Thus by developing the ability to become aware of, accept, symbolize, and talk about feelings, reflect on them, and access and develop other more compassionate and coping parts of the self, vulnerable and distressed parts of the self are regulated and soothed. Working with emotion in therapy is thus analogous to the development of emotion regulation that occurs in the process of normal development. Sustained empathic attunement to clients' emotions and to the nuances of their experience becomes a crucial therapeutic task in helping people become aware of and regulate their emotional experience.

ACTIVATING EMOTIONAL SCHEMES IN THERAPY

Therapists thus work with emotion schemes in a variety of ways. For example, they may acknowledge and affirm current experience and help clients strengthen that which is adaptive and growth producing. Or they may help clients to symbolize in words that which is traumatic or maladaptive, thereby helping them assimilate and contain this material; they may facilitate working through and emotional completion through helping clients to reprocess painful emotional experience; or they may restructure the maladaptive schemes that produce bad feelings, thereby creating new self-experience and personal meaning.

Therapists activate emotion schemes within the context of a safe, empathic therapeutic environment. In addition to empathic attunement, appropriate degrees of stimulation or intensification are used at appropriate times to increase arousal and to prime the schemes for activation, allowing clients easier access to their experience.

In our work with emotion we use a process-oriented experiential approach (Greenberg et al., 1993). This approach is based on following the client's moment-by-moment emotional process. The key clinical decision for the therapist rests on what aspect of the moment-by-moment process to focus on. As a guide, the therapist must take account of many factors, the most significant of which is the emotional aliveness of the presented material. In our view those states of mind in which emotion is particularly vivid and poignant are the ones most highly related to the client's well-being.

It is useful to note that the emotion schemes that we are talking about are intermediate-level, situation-related models. They are not nearly as large as identities, life scripts, or relational themes, but they are also not as small as simple acts or thoughts. As any event is experienced, there is a brief envelope of time in which the experience can be symbolized in awareness or pass away unsymbolized. It is these micromoments of attending to and symbolizing our experience in awareness that are the fundamental acts of our construction of being-in-the-world. In addition to the micromomentary process of catching the fleeting moment in the present, we appear to segment our concrete experiences of these moments in memory into chunks of different duration. We thus tend to experience things in small units ranging from the single moment of "catching the look on her face" to an episode of a number of seconds, for example, experiencing "holding him while he cried" or "having a conversation yesterday about our children." It is these episodic chunks of experience that need to be worked with in therapy (Korman & Greenberg, 1996). In this approach it is the shifting moment-by-moment activation and synthesis of schemes, in ongoing interaction with the other, that is viewed as determining experience, not a trait or global template like a core conflict, a role-relationship theme, or a core belief. It is thus these shifting experienced meanings and interactions, either of the remembered past or of the present moment, that become the focus of therapy.

Therapy is thus a process of schemes being activated both by self-generated internal processes and through interactions with the therapist. New schemes continue to be activated by the ever-changing present through dialogue with the therapist. This occurs as much through nonverbal emotional cues such as the melody and tempo of the the the therapist's voice, facial expressions, and general manner as by what is said. Much therapy then consists of identifying important moments or events in the sessions in which key emotion schemes have been activated, and intervening at these moments in ways most appropriate to the activated states (Greenberg et al., 1993).

AFFECT, EMOTION, AND FEELING

In the history of scholarship concerning the concepts of affect, emotion, and feeling, no clear demarcation has been formulated about the use of the terms "affect," "emotion," and "feeling" themselves (Hillman, 1960; Jaspers, 1963; James, 1890/1950; Freud, 1915/1963). Izard (1979) has suggested that emotion is a combination of affective and intellectual processes, whereas feeling reflects an irreducible affective state that is usually enriched, only in retrospect, by meaning and rationale. Despite this lack of scholarly clarity, we find it helpful to distinguish between them in the following way:

1. *Affect* refers to an unconscious biological response to stimulation. It involves automatic, physiological, motivational, and neural processes involved in the evolutionary adaptive behavioral response system. Affects do not involve reflective evaluation. They just happen, whereas both emotions and feelings are conscious products of these unconscious affective processes.

2. *Feeling* involves awareness of the basic sensations of affect. This involves bodily felt experience such as "feeling shaky" or "feeling tense." The more complex bodily felt feelings that involve felt meaning, such as feeling "down" or humiliated, feeling that something is not right, or feeling that one doesn't care, we call *complex feelings*. These involve relating affect to one's view of oneself.

3. Consciously experienced human *emotions* are experiences that arise when action tendencies and feeling states are joined with evoking

situations and self. Emotions are thus experiences that involve the integration of many levels of processing (Greenberg & Safran, 1987). They include the experience of discrete emotions such as fear, anger, and sadness, which have specific action tendencies and facial expressions, as well as the more complex emotions such as jealousy and pride, which are more related to a complex story or script. Emotions give personal meaning to our experience.

INTEGRATING EMOTION AND REASON

While most theories of the therapeutic effects of emotion have traditionally emphasized the irrationality of emotion, we will argue for the organizing role of emotion, showing how emotions guide and enhance decision making and problem solving. Emotions inform us of what is of concern to us. They set goals for cognition and in so doing can be seen as setting problems for cognition to solve. In this book we will thus focus on the importance of working with emotion in therapy and of integrating it with reason to form new meaning.

Emotions arise out of a complex constructive process that synthesizes many levels of information processing (Barnard & Teasdale, 1991; Greenberg et al., 1993; Greenberg & Pascual-Leone, 1995; Teasdale & Bernard, 1993; Watson & Greenberg, 1995). Affective, cognitive, motivational, and sensorimotor sources of information are always being complexly synthesized. All help determine human experience and action. However, not only is there a tacit, ongoing synthesis of many levels of information processing that produces feeling, but once this is synthesized in awareness there is also a more conscious process of integrating emotion and reason. Emotions emerge into consciousness by attending to a bodily felt sense and symbolizing this in awareness. Consciously symbolized material to varying degrees is then reflected on to create new meaning and to aid problem solving and decision making.

Consciousness in this view is not at the top of the hierarchy of control of human experience, nor is it the sole player. Rather, the emotion scheme, a tacit emotional–motivational–cognitive level of experiential processing, is an important player. Emotion schemes form the highest level of processing, higher than conscious reasoning or automated behavior. This level of processing guides both conscious thought and action and provides us with our complex, emotionally toned sense of things (it is a bodily felt sense) that is crucial in guiding decision making and choice. It provides us with our sense of well-being, of "being on top of the world," or our sense of malaise, of "being down in the dumps." This high-level tacit level of processing is a highly personal integration of biology and experience and acts as a sophisticated source of information about ourselves in relation to the world. It is this tacit level of emotional–motivational–cognitive processing that governs consciousness (Greenberg et al., 1993).

EMOTION AND REASON IN EVOLUTION

Emotions serve as an ongoing base of consciousness. They are continually present at some level of intensity and are a fundamental source of organismic vitality. Human organisms evolved to be proactive as well as reactive, and a genetically determined, neurally based emotion-activation system evolved to keep the organism continually active, exploring, and creative (Izard, 1993). The positive emotions appear to have evolved to serve the purpose of keeping the organism proactively adaptive.

Evolution, however, has provided us with two basic information-processing systems—an emotionally based, experiential one, and a rationally based, conceptual one. It is the integration of these two that in the final analysis produces adaptive behavior. As one experiences feelings, one also often consciously reflects on them. People constantly organize their experience in particular ways, integrating their cultural learning with their emotional sense of being to create new meaning. It is crucial to recognize that two distinct levels of meaning production guide human functioning: the conscious conceptual and the tacit experiential. It is the integration of these two levels that leads to adaptive functioning.

If I wake up emotionally ready to face the day, I will tackle projects with enthusiasm and I will think positively about how to do this. If I awake afraid and depressed, my emotions signal that something is awry in the way in which I am conducting my life or that something has happened that requires my attention. Having attended to the emotional signal, I begin the process of consciously reflecting on my experience and reorganizing my world. In order to do this I need to be able to first tolerate my feelings, integrate them into my sense of self, attend to them, and use them as signals. Having received the signal that all is well, I proceed to action, or having received the signal that there is a problem, I begin to act with awareness to discover and create solutions to the problems that have produced the bad feeling. It is in this way that emotions motivate and guide actions and set problems for reason to solve.

STRUCTURE OF THE BOOK

This book is divided into three parts.

Part I lays out the theoretical foundations of emotion: Chapter 2 discusses the nature and function of emotion, as well as its sources and its regulation; Chapter 3 presents a scheme for the assessment of different types of emotion expression in therapy and discusses the need for differential intervention with different types of emotion; Chapter 4 discusses emotional disorder and distinguishes between the role of emotional pain and bad feelings in dysfunction.

Part II lays out the intervention framework and the principles of emotionally focused intervention. This part begins with a discussion in Chapter 5 of the processes of change in an emotionally focused approach to treatment. Next, Chapter 6 presents the principles and three phases of treatment, thus serving as a type of manual of this approach.

In Part III, we focus on descriptions of and clinical work with the different emotions of anger (Chapter 7), sadness and distress (Chapter 8), fear and anxiety (Chapter 9), shame (Chapter 10), and the more pleasant emotions of love, interest/excitement, and joy (Chapter 11). The book concludes with a discussion of the training of therapists to work with emotion (Chapter 12). In this last chapter we emphasize that training needs to include both experiential work and development of perceptual, conceptual, interventive, and relational skills.

PART ONE

THEORETICAL FRAMEWORK

CHAPTER TWO

What Is Emotion?

*I*N THIS CHAPTER we will describe some basic features of emotion. We will show how emotion is fundamentally adaptive. In addition we will show that basic emotions are best characterized by those experiences in which the organism is bodily aroused and prepared for action. We also will demonstrate that human beings not only have emotions but also need to learn, by various means, to regulate their emotionality. We will suggest, too, that complex, emotionally toned experience is developed from basic emotions. This occurs as an individual's ability to synthesize, symbolize, and regulate this increasingly complex source of information and action grows. Finally, we will describe how this tacit synthesis results in a high-level form of knowing—our bodily felt sense of things and our personal meanings.

We can see the interplay of these features in every case. For example, a woman in therapy who had been sexually abused as a child said, "I feel like part of me is still a little girl, but I am almost afraid of that little girl." This feeling—"afraid of that little girl"—expressed a complex, felt meaning filled with significance. In response to the therapist's empathic exploration of this fear—"Something about her scares you?"—the client began to talk about how dirty, worthless, and ashamed she felt, and how she pulled away from this part of herself, afraid that if others knew this part they would reject her. This attention to, and exploration of, her feeling afraid helped identify the problem of feeling ashamed and worthless and established a focus for treatment. Thus feeling "almost afraid" of the little girl involved a complex meaning and tendency to pull away from the experience, an action that was probably adaptive in its original context but now resulted in her isolation from her self and others.

EMOTIONS ORGANIZE US FOR ACTION

Emotions regulate mental functioning, organizing both thought and action. First, they establish goal priorities and organize us for particular actions (Frijda, 1986). Thus fear sets a goal for escape and readies us for flight; anger sets the goal for overcoming obstacles and readies us for attack. The goals they prompt are largely related to the regulation of our social bonds. Happiness and love, for example, provide for cooperation; sadness, for withdrawal or help seeking; and anger, for boundary management. Second, emotions set the goals toward which cognitions and action strive, making affect a crucial determiner of human conduct (Frijda, 1986; Oatley & Jenkins, 1992; Pascual-Leone, 1990a, 1990b, 1991). Someone who is sad and in need of comfort will find his or her perceptions and actions influenced in a number of ways. For example, one person will begin to move toward comfort; another will begin to think more and more sadness-enhancing thoughts such as "I'm all alone, no one cares" or will begin to retrieve sad memories and yearn for contact, comfort, and companionship. The first person, who has enjoyed good attachments with significant others and so learned that comfort is possible, will eventually reach out and make contact with others. For those like the second person, above, who have learned that needs are not met, resignation, which is the poison of action, sets in. They quickly feel, "It's no use, I never get what I need," and give up. Here thought and action are unable to be mobilized in the service of goal attainment. Thus emotion sets the desired *end goal;* cognition and learning provides the *means* whereby the goal is met or not met. Emotions therefore are the guiding structures of our lives especially in our relations with others. Cognition thus sets out to solve the problem of how to reach the emotion-set goal of connecting, of getting comfort, or of separating.

Recent developments in neuroscience suggest that the emotional processing of simple sensory features occurs extremely early in the processing sequence that produces emotional reactions. Stimuli arrive as inputs via a special path to the subcortical areas of the brain that deal with emotion (the amygdala and the thalamus) prior to the construction, in the neocortex, of real-world objects and events from the same simple sensory stimuli. According to LeDoux (1993), this initial "precognitive" emotional processing is highly adaptive because it enables us to respond quickly to important events without having to wait for more complex and time-consuming processing. It may not be in our best interest, for example, to spend extra, precious time identifying a loud approaching noise from the forest as to its source—it is better to act first and think later. Likewise, it is better to jump back quickly from a sinuous-looking form in the forest only to discover later by means of more thorough conscious analysis that it is a circular branch not a snake.

The brain rapidly preconsciously appraises situations as, say, strange or dangerous, and sets off affect alarms that direct cognition to search for and identify the unfamiliar, evaluate the danger, and plan action. The emotional centers of the brain receive and process input earlier than do the planning and decision-making centers, which by the time they process the same input have already been oriented toward it in a particular way by information from the emotional centers. Essentially, again affect sets problems for cognitions to solve (Damasio, 1994; LeDoux, 1994; Pascual-Leone, 1991). Emotion, then, is fundamentally about motivation and action, setting goals and readying the person for action, whereas cognition is fundamentally about knowledge and involves analyzing the situation and deciding on action (Izard, 1993). Emotion initially preceded cognition in motivating action, but in our present evolutionary stage it is virtually impossible to experience emotion without cognitive functioning. Emotion essentially tells us what is of concern to us and organizes us for action, but thinking or reason is needed to further analyze the situation, to validate or correct our automatic appraisals and apprehensions of pattern, and to plan and decide what actions to actually execute. In the context of the vast cultural evolution of the last centuries, it increasingly seems that it is the integration of emotion and reason that results in the most adaptive response. We need emotion to tell us what is of concern to us and to set a goal to be attained, and we need cognition to help make sense of our experience and reason to help us figure out the best way to achieve the goal or satisfy the concern in our specific cultural context.

EMOTIONS ARE FUNDAMENTALLY ADAPTIVE

Emotions, then, are neither rational nor irrational; rather, they are *adaptive* (Darwin, 1872/1955). They are internal signals directing us to sustain life. In comparison with cognition, emotion is a biologically older, adaptive, rapid-action system, a system designed to enhance survival. A principal function of emotion is to connect our biological nature with the world within which it is embedded. Emotions respond immediately to the survival-related truth of things. Emotion regulates attention, monitoring the environment for adaptation-relevant events and alerting consciousness when they arise. Fear thus warns us of danger; disgust turns us away from decay; and compassion enables us to respond to another's pain. Different emotions alert us to different things and serve distinctly different functions. Some feelings, such as anger and fear, warn us of danger, whereas others, such as sadness and love, move us toward people; yet others, such as shame and guilt, warn us of internal dis-ease; and the joyously positive feelings enhance life and promote the pursuit of happiness. There is considerable evidence that emotion serves psychologically adaptive functions at an early age (Frijda, 1986; Izard, 1990; Thompson, 1988). As well as being adaptively *self*-regulating, emotions are adaptively *other*-regulating, such as when the cry of distress brings comforting others toward us or when the display of anger pushes impinging others away.

The adaptive function of emotions is better understood when we look at the differences in the so-called positive and negative emotions. Here "positive" and "negative" refer to the phenomenological aspect of emotion, that is, to our general experience of the emotion as pleasant or unpleasant, rather than to its adaptive function, which is positive by definition. The positively experienced emotions are crucial in motivating proactive exploratory behavior. Interest and excitement are an essential element in promoting exploration and novel behavior and are an essential aspect of our being growth-oriented, adaptive organisms. Joy and happiness, which result both from contact with an attachment figure and from a sense of efficacy, also serve to keep the organism proactive, continually seeking attachments and mastery. Those positive emotions that have their own specific adaptive action tendency are few in number, however, involving joy, interest, and the complex feeling of caring or love. We often just feel generally good, and this response—most like a mild feeling of joy—keeps us open, curious, and active rather than leading to more differentiated specific actions.

In therapy it is the positive emotions, especially interest and curiosity, that are helpful in motivating people to explore further their inner worlds, and of course the positive emotions are crucial in motivating them to explore the world outside of therapy and to make new connections and try new behaviors. In addition to broadening options for action, positive emotions often act as antidotes to negative emotions. They restore balance in physiological responses and rid people of the action tendency set up by the negative emotions. Thus joy or love speeds the recovery from sadness.

In sharp contrast to the small number of basic positive emotions, there is a large repertoire of negative emotions (Ekman & Friesen, 1975). Feelings like fear, despair, anger, shame, and disgust all can preoccupy us, but none would be mistaken for the others. We appear to have evolved more and more differentiated negative emotions to help us in our quest for survival. Each has its own action tendency.

Anger impels us toward an antagonist or annoyance—and, in extremes, we want to lash out at or attack the object of our fury. In fear, we shrink away from something sensed as threatening and want to escape it. Sadness closes us down, and we want to hide under the covers and shut out the world. Disgust leads us to expel unwanted intrusions. In evolutionary terms, whereas the positive emotions were necessary for enhancing life, it appears that they did not have to differentiate into as many kinds of signals as did the negative emotions. It is the negative emotions that have evolved to prepare us for dealing with numerous different potentially harmful situations by means of many types of responses. Given that emotions provide us with feedback about our reactions to situations and provide rapid-action tendencies to promote survival, it is of crucial importance to adaptation that we attend to our feelings. All the primary emotions are useful and serve adaptive purposes. They are not bad intrusions to be prevented, nor are they toxic substances to be discharged or got rid of.

Whether emotions are automatically or deliberatively generated, they lead to actions designed to change the organism–environment relationship so as to make the emotion no longer necessary. Thus when I cry I increase the probability of receiving comfort from self and other, when I'm angry I increase the probability of chasing the other away, and when I'm afraid I increase the probability of escaping. Once the goals of comfort, assertion, or escape have been achieved, the emotional response is no longer necessary and abates. This is the value of expressing previously avoided emotion in therapy. When the emotion is expressed to a responsive therapist it has an opportunity to shift into something else, to evolve. Clients experience a sense of relief after having a good cry, especially with a receptive therapist, and fully expressed and validated anger can quickly shift to sadness and vice versa.

The *primary* emotions are all characterized by their adaptive action tendencies, which are designed to change the organism's relationship with the environment. This is done not by changing the environment but by changing the self. Thus in anger we puff up and become larger, thrusting forward; in fear we shrink away; in sadness we lower our eyes and close down, whereas interest and happiness open us up to the world. In therapy it is important to help clients attend to these bodily experiences. Taking this internal focus rather than focusing on changing the environment can be self-empowering. For example, clients who stop themselves from expressing their sadness and loss, or their anger at violation, through such injunctions as "What's the use, I'll never get what I want anyway," need to experience what it is like to give voice to their own sadness or assert the right to express anger whether the other responds or not. Feeling entitled to one's sadness or anger empowers by changing one's internal sense of self. This internal change enabling one to accept feelings translates into a new confidence and strength and a more contactful relationship with the environment.

EMOTIONS INFLUENCE MEMORY AND THOUGHT

Emotion also influences cognition in a variety of other ways. Affect can be experienced in consciousness as unlabeled, unarticulated feeling states such as irritability or happiness, and moods such as these have been shown to influence what people remember, think, and do (Blaney, 1986; Isen, 1984).

Feelings and emotions also exert a powerful influence on reason. They can enhance or impair reason and decision making. They enhance decision making by helping determine the significance to self of particular outcomes. They help to reduce one's options by rapidly and preconsciously appraising things as good or bad for oneself. Thus in trying to decide what university to go to or when to make an appointment, emotional preferences help to limit our options to those universities we like or times that are more convenient for us. The emotion system thus provides "gut" feelings about things to guide us. These feelings also help us focus attention on negative possibilities and provide an immediate response that steers us away from them. A rational analysis of the situation follows, but only after the automatic affective appraisal has rapidly reduced options. This increases the accuracy and efficiency of decision making.

Brain-damaged patients who do not have a bodily felt or intuitive ("gut") feeling but whose rational functioning remains fully intact are severely impaired in real life decision-making situations that are dynamic and multidimensional (Damasio, 1994). They do not have an intuitive sense to guide their rational thinking and to signify that some things are more important than others. They therefore become stuck in pondering all possibilities. Emotions therefore clearly influence cognition and action and are essential to real-life decision making. In psychotherapy clients who try to intellectually resolve decisional conflicts (Greenberg & Webster, 1982), such as choosing or separating from a partner or deciding on a course of action, without attending to their felt preferences go around and around on the merry-go-round of pros and cons and are unable to decide. Attending to gut feelings adds weight to options and has to be attended to in therapy in order for a decision to crystallize or new meaning to emerge.

Recently Bernet (1995) developed a measure of three perceptual styles people used in processing their bodily feelings. A person with a body-based style perceives emotions through an integrated awareness of subtle physical changes. This style correlates with established measures of mental health as well as with warmth, aesthetic feelings, and life satisfaction. A style with an emphasis on evaluation is more introspective, interpreting feelings cognitively as if from an outside perspective. This style correlates with neuroticism, vigilance, apprehension, tension, and discontent. Finally, a style of looking to logic uses reasoning to understand and control feelings. This style shows no correlation with mental health but correlates negatively with warmth. This work suggests that limited awareness of body cues in mediating between reactions and emotions may be a component of neuroticism, and that awareness of subcortically generated, bodily felt experience and the ability to perceive subtle feelings may optimize mental health and improve personal functioning.

EMOTIONS ARE MOTIVATIONAL

Emotional responses, through their physiological and action tendency components, prepare and motivate people to deal with emotion-eliciting events. In addition, emotions are often sought after as their own rewards, thereby motivating behavior to increase the probability of occurrence of the behaviors that produce certain emotional states. Emotions are therefore both ends in themselves (states we desire to achieve or avoid) and the means of guiding us toward those ends (dispositions to act). Fear, as we have said, is aversive, thereby motivating escape or avoidance, and simultaneously provides physiological and motor responses to support flight. Joy is both pleasant (thereby motivating its attainment) while simultaneously providing physiological and motor responses to support opening up and approach. Children from birth are motivated by ongoing efforts to preserve a sense of emotional well-being. Adults in therapy are constantly striving toward feeling better. It is this tendency and the moment-by-moment process of evaluating what is good for one that needs to be focused on in therapy and in life. This is done by attending to feelings to guide our actions.

Living *in* the present by attending to our complex felt sense of what is good for us, however, is not the same as living *for* the present, which involves simply doing what feels good, regardless of the consequence. This latter process lacks the subtlety of attending to our complex felt sense that integrates the past, present, and future in favor of attending only to the strongest momentary impulse. Thus living "in the present" is not to be confused with living "for the present."

EMOTIONS INFORM US

Emotions give us information about our reactions to situations. Much emotion results from automatic evaluations of the significance of situations for our well-being. They result from appraisals of the relevance of situations to our concerns (Frijda, 1986). This organismic process of tacitly evaluating what is good or bad for us is often referred to as feeling. Emotions are attended to, to tell us how we are reacting to situations. It is important to be aware that we are afraid and are organized to flee. Second, and equally important, emotions that are explored give us access to our appraisals of the situation and our currently operating needs and goals (Greenberg & Korman, 1993). Identifying idiosyncratic appraisals and needs forms a primary focus of therapeutic work. Thus a client who feels angry and is able to differentiate this into "I feel angry because it's so unfair" begins to clarify that he feels unjustly treated and wishes for fair play. Another client, who articulates that she feels "angry because I never know when he's going to be there for me," is able to discern that she appraises her husband as abandoning her and that her concern is for support and predictability.

EMOTION IS COMMUNICATION

Emotions provide information to others about our intentions or our readiness to act. In evolutionary terms, as primary signaling systems, emotions enhanced survival. Infants' cries brought their caretakers toward them, whereas angry snarls showed hostile intentions, thereby often providing the possibility of avoiding violent conflict.

   In interpersonal relationships the constant sending and reading of signals about emotional states, especially through the face, greatly informs and regulates interaction (Greenberg & Johnson, 1988). In intimate relationships being perceptive or sensitive to our partners' states can save us a lot of difficulty. Being on the receiving end of our partners' sensitivity to our emotional states can make us feel very cared for. When we feel our partner is oblivious to us we can feel quite neglected. Clients in therapy understand implicitly that if they change themselves emotionally on the inside, this will be conveyed on the outside and others will treat them differently. If they feel more confident, they will be able to assertively express themselves. If they are less fearful, they will be more able to get jobs and be treated with respect.

SOURCES OF EMOTION

Emotions originate from many sources—neurochemical, physiological, biopsychological, and cognitive (Izard, 1991, 1993). An important psychological process involved in the generation of emotion, and one that is of great relevance to psychotherapy, is the process in which emotion results from a person's automatic appraisal of a situation, first in relation to a need/goal/concern, and then in relation to a coping ability (Frijda, 1986; Lazarus, 1986). For example, in a situation involving an important loss, sadness tells us of the need for the lost object. Adaptive sadness will run its course as long as the person perceives that he or she is able to heal from the loss and move on. However, sadness turns into chronic depression if the person feels hopeless about ever healing, or it turns into anxiety if the person anticipates impending danger and threat to safety as a result of the loss.

Appraisals can be both rapid and automatic, making emotion a biologically adaptive rapid-action response, as well as slow and deliberate, making emotion a culturally and socially based consequence of reflection and decision making. Immediacy of response appears to vary with the intensity of the current experience and of associated past experiences. Thus, if in the past one has had severe experiences of being criticized, humiliated, or abandoned in situations relevant to self-esteem or attachment, one becomes sensitive or hypersensitive to cues that this might occur. The relevant pattern of cues is vigilantly (and unconsciously) scanned for, rapidly and tacitly appraised, and results in a feeling of vulnerability. Most often fear, shame, or sadness is what makes the person feel attacked, mocked, or dismissed, and the thoughts maintain and intensify the feeling rather than produce it. Conscious appraisals such as "I have been wronged" thus often follow or accompany rather than produce the feeling, in this case anger.

Under circumstances not involving high stress or personal vulnerability, emotional experience is mediated by slower, higher-level cognitive evaluation and is less reactive, such as when you consciously realize you disagree with someone or appraise that your amorous advances are not being received. On a conscious level, you feel challenged or rebuffed and then decide how to deal with the situation. Whether or not you have the capacity to deal with the disagreement or the rejection will make you feel either confident or threatened. In therapy, we most often deal more with the rapidly activated responses.

Emotion is thus activated by a variety of sources, including conscious and nonconscious, as well as cognitive and noncognitive, sources. Much therapeutically relevant emotion is activated by the automatic recognition of complex patterns, not by conscious thoughts, and is more like apprehension than reasoning. The way people apprehend or frame events depends on their needs/goals/concerns and values. We thus often respond powerfully to a look on a face or a gesture, and without conscious appraisal apprehend disapproval because we are concerned with getting approval.

Emotionally focused therapy (EFT) does not concentrate on exploring the automatic thought that supposedly preceded the reaction, but rather focuses on exploring the bodily felt sense and action tendency forming the response. Focusing on the emotion-generating processes and unpacking the complex tacit meanings and network of associations helps get at the feeling and the need or goal prompting the reaction. Semantic representations such as thoughts often are the product of complex emotional and cognitive activity rather than the basis of it. Thus, what needs to be explored are the bodily experience, situational cues, memories, needs, goals, expectations, and the person's sense of efficacy that lead to the thoughts, rather than the thoughts themselves.

EMOTIONAL EXPERIENCE

Much emotional experience occurs in the form of complex feelings and meanings, such as feeling humiliated or awkward or feeling "over the hill" or "washed out" (Gendlin, 1962, 1974). These feelings are generated automatically by organizations of experience that we have called emotion schemes (Greenberg et al., 1993). These schemes are complex internal organizations of different degrees of sensation, physiology, emotion memory, and situational cues and their meanings, as well as rules or beliefs learned as the person develops (Greenberg & Safran, 1987, 1989; Leventhal, 1982, 1984). These emotion schemes, which integrate many levels of information processing, incorporate our emotional learning history and constitute our most fundamental level of processing. They develop into new fundamental sources for automatic, bodily felt, "instinctive" feeling reactions. These schemes and their ongoing dynamic syntheses provide a new higher-level "intuitive sense" of things that we appropriately value highly and that act as prereflective guides to our behavior. They are an organized synthesis of our biology, our psychology, and our culture. They capture very-high-level patterns or regularities in experience and provide a complex meaning-generating structure that evaluates the significance of situations for our well-being and, by apprehending patterns, provide holistic meanings.

These internal structures and their apprehending process provide us with an inner valuing process that is superior to our intellect alone. This is because they integrate information from both representational and sensory levels of processing and are therefore our richest level of information processing. It is important here to distinguish between the operation of purely cognitive *schemas,* which are representational in nature and inform us of the truth of something in a conscious conceptual way, and emotion *schemes.* The latter fundamentally are not representational but are action and experience producing. They inform us of the value of things to us, generating experience in a sensory, bodily felt manner and organizing us for action. The complexly synthesized feelings produced by emotion schemes tell us what is important to us in our lives, and it is these bodily felt meanings that guide thought and action. They provide meaning and, in telling us the value of things to us, add emotional meaning to our lives. Sensing and thinking tell us only so much about our world: sensing tells us what is there, and thinking helps establish what is true or false. Feelings, however, add evaluations of what is good and bad and what is significant to our well-being. The organism comes into the world with a basic set of built-in affective preferences in relation to survival. Under the influence of experience these expand exponentially, providing us with a basis for the creation of complex personal meanings.

It is important to note that many of these culturally influenced, complex feelings, such as feeling jealous, fragile, or "on top of things," do not have specific action tendencies, nor are they characterized by unique facial expressions. They occur more as bodily experienced feelings. The more complex discrete emotions involve a story or script and *judgments* rather than action tendencies that distinguish them apart. Thus moral emotions such as pride, envy, and jealousy are complex feelings based on culturally ascribed values, and they involve complex judgments about well-being, about agents, and about proper actions (Frijda, 1986). Feelings or bodily felt meanings are the not yet clearly symbolized syntheses of all of our complex internal reactions (Greenberg & Pascual-Leone, 1995, 1996). These complex syntheses then become the basis for a set of symbolized feelings such as feeling complete or feeling shattered, which provide us with a high-level sense of what is significant to us and personally meaningful.

For example, a client who had ongoing struggles with her ex-husband over issues concerning their two children entered therapy depressed, in despair at her ex-husband's coldness and distance toward her. Since he had a new family, he had put their children "on the shelf." It was easy for this client to be angry at her ex-husband, and she had legitimate concerns that needed to be acknowledged and validated, but there also appeared to be much reactive anger to unacknowledged underlying feelings. More central emotions seemed to be how much it hurt her to see her children feeling neglected, rejected, and cast aside. As cues of hurt and sadness about the children and her wants appeared in therapy, the therapist directed her attention to this internal experience, validated the client's experience about her children, but also helped focus her on her own losses. Her painful experience was aroused by the therapist saying, "It hurts deeply to see them cast aside, cuts you to the core." When the client responded that she "can't stand it that they think their father doesn't love them," the therapist reflected that she can't stand to think of them hurting and empathically conjectures that it "probably evokes some profound losses of your own." This accessed the client's sadness about her losses in the marriage, how she herself felt cast aside, rejected—all the things she had missed since the marriage ended.

In exploring her experience it became evident that these losses had not been grieved over by her because she was the one who chose to leave the marriage. She felt that she had no right to grieve. One of the ways she stopped herself from fully acknowledging her loss was through internalized injunctions such as "You made your bed, now you sleep in it." The therapist attended to signs of her underlying primary sadness: "Sounds like part of you would still like to be close." The client agreed that, yes, she would like to be friends but that she had no right to expect that under the circumstances. The therapist replied, "Perhaps it's not realistic to expect, but it sounds like part of you still wants it." This helped the client reframe her reactive anger. Having her experience validated helped the client symbolize her desire for support, friendship, partnership, and appreciation of her parenting, and to share joys and sorrows concerning the children. The therapist responded that it is "hard to be alone in parenting" and that there "must have been many times you wanted to share stuff with him." This helped the client acknowledge the loss of these hopes and dreams to grieve for the lost friendship, evoking tears for her own loneliness. This therapeutic weeping (and self-awareness) led to completion of her grieving and to a restructuring of the emotion scheme related to loss of her marriage.

Thus the client was able to reduce some of her unresolved feelings toward her husband. She created a new narrative of her experience, reinterpreting her reactions as coming from a place of loss and sadness rather than simply anger, and was able to speak from that experience with her ex-husband. She could be less defensive and more open about what the loss of the marriage meant to her, acknowledging its value and dignity, and then carry that self-awareness into a new relationship with her ex-husband. These feelings were all complex syntheses of many aspects of her experience, and as she symbolized them and reflected on them they changed to new complex feelings.

TRUSTING OUR EMOTIONS

If complex feelings and the more primary emotions stem from a fundamentally adaptive system, are we proposing that feelings and emotions are always to be trusted? This is a complex issue to which our answer is a definite "possibly." It depends on what feelings are to be trusted and in what way: trusted blindly to determine action—no; trusted as primary sources of information about our reactions and about what we experience—absolutely! Given this feeling, we then need to reflect on the best course of action to enhance our well-being.

In the final analysis, we are our feelings and how we deal with them. Feeling is the process of being. Passions are so called because they capture the automaticity of feelings—we passively receive them. Our contention is that attempts to not receive our feelings is one of the greatest follies of the active, controlling orientation of the Western mind. Rather, we need to live in mindful harmony with our feelings, not attempt to control them. However, rather than suggesting that we surrender and be governed only by emotions, we are suggesting an integration of will, intellect, desire, and emotion into a holistic response of the self. We need to integrate our heads and our hearts, being neither compelled by emotion nor cut off from it. Emotion is not opposed to reason. Emotions guide and manage thought in fundamental ways and complement the deficiencies of thinking. They make best courses of action possible when rational decision making is not possible because of partial knowledge, conflicting aims, and limited resources (Oatley, 1992).

In order to trust our emotions we have to handle them with a special kind of wisdom or intelligence. Emotional intelligence (Salovey, Hsee, & Mayer, 1993) involves knowing our emotions and being self-aware. This entails recognizing our feelings as they arise, as well as being able to manage them to effect our aims. Being aware helps each of us handle feelings so that they do not overwhelm, and helps us soothe ourselves and manage our anxiety, anger, and sadness. Emotional intelligence also involves being able to control impulses and to be able to motivate ourselves. Being able to defer our emotional responses and reflect on them is quintessentially human. Finally emotional intelligence entails the ability to recognize emotions in others and thereby to handle relationships successfully (Salovey et al., 1993). All these abilities emerge from emotion awareness, the bedrock of emotional intelligence. Culturally appropriate expression of emotion has become more and more important as culture has become more complex. This requires awareness of both one's own emotional reactions and the social context, and the ability to integrate these into a reasoned course of action.

Therapy thus needs to build awareness of emotion as a first step to better adaptation. For example, a client who had grown up in an environment in which her mother's anger was out of control and destructive had learned to be afraid of all her own feelings, especially her anger. Instead of feeling the variety of her feelings and being able to use them as a guide in her life, she chronically collapsed into hurt, depression, and powerlessness. She had great difficulties establishing firm interpersonal boundaries. The therapist began by validating her fear of her anger, understanding how, having witnessed the destructiveness of her mother's anger, she saw anger as destructive. In discussing the client's anger, however, the therapist distinguished between reactive, out-of-control anger and healthy, adaptive anger, the type that facilitates boundary setting and standing up for ourselves. The therapist then helped the client access memories of situations in which her mother was abusive. In response to this memory the client, in the session, felt a flicker of anger toward her mother at such unfair treatment. While the memory was alive, the therapist, who was attuned to markers of the client's habitual collapsing into powerlessness and hurt encouraged her to resist this collapse and rather to stay with her righteous anger. She was encouraged to acknowledge her anger, to put her feet flat on the floor, and to speak from this position of power. The client said to her imagined mother, "It's not right what you did, it's not fair. I did not deserve that treatment." Here the client became aware of and began to express her anger. Other feelings soon followed.

EMOTION AS PROCESS

Feelings and emotions involve a natural process of emergence and completion. This spontaneous process of arising and passing away occurs because many feelings involve an automatic apprehending process over which we have little conscious control. To some degree, we can control what we feel by limiting our exposure to external evoking cues or by trying to control our conscious thoughts, but we can do little to prevent the automatic evocation of many feelings. They result from complex preconscious processes of apprehension, by a sensing of things that precedes any form of conscious symbolic thought (Greenberg & Safran, 1987; Zajonc, 1980). Given that people cannot control these affective experiences, they had best learn to accept their feelings and learn from them.

The natural process of feeling can be depicted as a set of phases (shown in Figure 2.1), those of emergence, awareness, owning, expressive action, and completion, followed again by the emergence of a new feeling, thereby beginning the cycle again. It is when this process is chronically interfered with—when, for example, emergence or identification is prevented, or experience is not symbolized in awareness, or expression is constantly interrupted and action and completion are repeatedly blocked—that people become stuck in a chronic bad feeling and become dysfunctional and chronically distressed.

One of the things we teach clients is to develop an attitude of openness and acceptance to feelings and to their mutative nature: feelings come and go, arise and pass away, and change over time. This helps people learn to integrate "unwanted" feelings, and not get stuck in particular feelings that can become pathological (Greenberg, 1995). For example, a client who had just received her divorce papers said she recognized this was important and sad but she felt flat. The therapist helped her overcome her avoidance by asking her to talk about what she had lost and what she missed. By attending to her sadness at losing the relationship she had had, and experiencing this more fully, she made a shift. She was able to distinguish that she no longer wanted the relationship as it now was, and she accepted that the relationship of the past was no more. She then felt that she could accept the end of the relationship because it was no longer a type of relationship of her choosing and was no longer good for her.

In accepting feelings it is important to recognize that feelings, although enhancing readiness to act, are not behaviors. Thus feeling angry or annoyed is not the same as being aggressive. Feelings imply that one sensorially experiences and is organized for particular actions, whereas behaving implies that one acts in the world. Feelings are subjective experience; behaviors are overt and subject to social regulation. Problems emerge when feelings and behaviors are confused. When people attempt to make their feelings rather than their behaviors

Emergence ➡Awareness ➡ Owning ➡ Expressive action ➡ Completion

FIGURE 2.1. The process of feeling.

conform to social norms, they begin to get involved in unhealthy self-manipulation and self-coercion. In order for people to deal with unwanted feelings, rather than trying to control them, they need to become aware of what they are doing that is keeping them stuck in the feeling, how they are interrupting the natural process of emergence and completion.

EMOTION REGULATION

From infancy, the child both experiences emotions and learns to regulate them (Thompson, 1990; Sroufe, 1996). Emotions energize, organize, and motivate adaptive functioning, but this depends on a variety of diverse processes by which emotion is regulated. Infants have the capacity to self-regulate experience, even if only rudimentarily. For example, they suck their thumbs in order to soothe themselves, or they cry to signal distress and evoke soothing responses from others. Emotion experience is initially primarily regulated by caretakers, but over the course of normal development it becomes increasingly self-regulated as a result of development in neurophysiology, cognition, language, and self-understanding. As children grow, the development of emotion-regulation skills is essential in helping organize emotive processes into the adaptive control of behavior.

The first aspect of affect regulation or self-organization is the process by which the basic neurochemical affective processes, physiological arousal, and expressive–motor processes are integrated into a coherent pattern. Over time this pattern of experience is experienced as a feeling and finally symbolized in awareness to provide an emotion such as anger or sadness. This is the most basic form of affect regulation—synthesizing raw affect into a coherent recognized pattern.

The development of emotion regulation can be seen as one of the major developmental tasks in the personal and interpersonal domain. To learn to regulate emotions in a healthy manner is a task that takes many years of practice. The development of emotion regulation is influenced by both internal and external factors. Beginning virtually from birth, developmental changes in the child's neurophysiological functioning provides greater stability in, and inhibitory control of, emotion. The development of cognitive and self-reflective capacities soon come to assist in the regulatory process. In addition, external influences on emotion regulation occur virtually from birth and continue even after regulation has been achieved. The newborn infant cannot consistently regulate emotional arousal without the assistance of caregivers and frequently becomes overaroused and disorganized.

The development of emotion regulation can be seen as a joint endeavor between infant and caretaker, and as involving a persistent coregulatory endeavor on behalf of the individual and the social environment throughout life.

Infants' emotional systems are involved in rapid evaluation of what is good or bad for them. Thus infants, right from birth, experience feelings and, as soon as they can construct schemes of sufficient complexity (Pascual-Leone, 1991), they use these feelings to construct a conscious personal sense of self. A major determinant of this self-construction is their intersubjective experience associated with their own automatic emotional reactions. An individual's sense of self is primordially organized around emotional schemes formed in primary attachment relationships. Affect regulation develops with maturation but also with the way caretakers react to the child's emotions; these experiences determine the affectively based sense of self. The views of others about one's emotional experience are synthesized with one's own internal experience to form emotion schematic records of self and circumstance. These emotional schemes become the core structures of the person and guide further growth. How one symbolizes one's internal states evolves in an intersubjective manner, and the "I" comes to see itself as a particular "me." This is mediated through others' views of, and responses to, the self (Guidano, 1987, 1995; Stern, 1985).

Emotional development is the story of the development of self-regulation—starting with the ability to internalize the soothing of the caretaker, to learning to suck one's thumb, to the use of a transitional object, to whistling in the dark to regulate one's fears, to the adult ability to ask for support when needed. These are the skills of growing to a sense of secure interdependence that is the sign of healthy emotion regulation. As a consequence of increased emotion regulation, whereas the infant may cry uncontrollably, the toddler can seek help and nurture, the preschooler can label and talk about feelings, and the school-age child can reflect on feelings and use deliberate ways of reducing distress and anxiety such as redirecting attention. The adolescent and adult then develop much greater self-understanding and much more complex and idiosyncratic ways of regulating emotion (some adaptive and others dysfunctional). Children's emotion-regulation strategies have been grouped into three categories: social support from either caregivers or peers; affect communication (of distress or anger); and autonomous regulation (distraction/avoidance or self-calming) (Kopp, 1989; Rossman, 1992). Distraction/avoidance and expressing of emotion to others have been found to be the least effective means of reducing children's vulnerability and enhancing self-esteem. The mature capacity to regulate internal states of emotional arousal, including their expression in productive and complex ways, is a crucial step toward adaptive and sophisticated functioning in adulthood. The ability to self-soothe (by internalizing the soothing of others) is crucial to development and stability, as is the ability to seek out caregivers' soothing.

Once the initial developmental task of synthesizing affect into emotional experience is achieved, the next level of regulation involves a self-organizing process. This process is the development of the person's relationship with his or her own emotional experience, either acknowledging it, accepting it, or disowning it. Even though human beings are born with biologically adaptive emotions, their adaptive functions are largely dependent on the ability to be aware of their emotions, to consciously experience specific emotions as signals for specific reactions. Thus the degree to which emotion serves an organizing or a disorganizing effect is dependent on the degree to which emotion is integrated into awareness. Thus emotions are not only activated but also need to be brought into awareness, differentiated, reflected on, and expressed in a socially appropriate manner.

Monsen (1994) has specified and developed a measure of four aspects of "affect consciousness": degree of awareness, affect tolerance (experiencing ability), nonverbal expressiveness, and conceptual expressiveness. He argues that it is important to be conscious of emotion and that awareness determines the degree to which the specific emotions will have an organizing or disorganizing effect on the person's ability to relate to self and others. A generally low degree of affect consciousness implies that the signal function of emotion will be deficient, motives for action will be vague, and there will be a loss of contact with a basic sense of self. Using this instrument, Monsen demonstrates significant positive correlations between global level of affect consciousness (an integration of the above four components) and measures of good functioning, such as global mental health, ego strength, and quality of interpersonal relationships. He demonstrates significant negative correlations with measures of maladaptive functioning, such as neuroticism, identity diffusion, and general symptomatology. These findings support the idea that emotion awareness is associated with personal and social adaptation and that integration of emotion is a key form of emotion regulation.

Once primitive affective experience is symbolized and integrated into one's view of self and thereby regulated, it is the *expression* of emotion that then involves regulation. Neither unbridled expression nor uncontrolled restraint is particularly healthy or adaptive. It is the ability to choose when to express one's emotions rather than to have one's emotions automatically control one's behavior that is ultimately adaptive. It is important to possess one's emotions rather than be possessed by them—to be master of one's passions rather than passion's slave. On the one hand, overcontrol and suppression of emotion is dysfunctional, both robbing people of their ability to orient themselves rapidly in their environments and producing internal stress. On the other hand, undercontrol and inability to regulate emotion can result in severe social disruption, often damaging interpersonal relations or hurting others as well as resulting in prolonged internal distress. The balanced ability to both have emotions and regulate them in contextually appropriate ways is the ultimate criterion of health.

Regulation of experience and expression affects the intensity of emotion, and it is often the intensity of emotion that determines its adaptiveness. Arousal is a valuable catalyst and organizer of behavior, but heightened arousal can be disorganizing and maladaptive. Again, it is the ability to achieve balance by regulating the intensity of emotional experience and its expression, either by automatic synthesizing processes or by conscious reflection, that is the ultimate goal and constitutes wisdom. There is a difference between having emotions and being overwhelmed by them. Feeling sad at the loss of a relationship is part of the process of breaking attachment bonds. Being overwhelmed with panic and despair by a rejection is not particularly adaptive. Generally, mild-to-moderate emotion appears to be most adaptive. Extreme emotions that erupt too intensely or last too long undermine our stability. Mild fear isn't distressing, can even be exciting, but terror is painful and disorganizing. Anger or indignation can promote assertiveness and effective action; loss of one's temper and rage can put one at a disadvantage. At times, however, intense anger or sadness are highly adaptive and appropriate, as are intense joy and love. It is when people are unable to regulate the intensity of emotions— are overwhelmed by them against their will such that they feel out of control—that problems arise.

In adulthood emotion regulation does not mean either control and suppression of expression or concealment of emotion from others, for the concealed or suppressed emotion still rages internally. Rather, it is the attainment of balanced experience and expression under one's aware control that is the goal. Affect needs to be regulated such that anxiety or rage does not run out of control. Emotions need to be recognized and translated into understandable messages and constructive action. In this way emotions are no longer purely reactive, but rather become a source of information about one's responses to situations.

Affective dysregulation is generally maladaptive. Our most primitive anger and fear responses were adaptive to the extreme dangers of the wild but are often out of place, in their original intensity, in the boardroom. Intense fear or rage in response to personal slights or rejections is dysfunctional, and this form of dysregulation leads to great personal distress. Wisdom and emotional maturity involves mastering the intensity of emotions so that they are experienced at their most adaptive levels. Emotional maturity also entails overcoming negative emotional learning so that past responses to present situations are not experienced in ways that are currently maladaptive. Adaptive socialization therefore requires the attainment of balance as opposed to the suppression of emotion. Peace and tranquility are attained in life by being able to experience current emotional reactions, to express one's feelings appropriately, to let the process run its course, to rise above the storm and inner turmoil of upsets of the past, and to overcome present maladaptive emotional reactions that occur as a function of past learning and internal conflict.

Emotional storms can overwhelm us, often as a result of prior emotional crises in which the emergency response has become laid down as the habitual one. In these situations the ability to regulate or calm oneself has been lost. These storms appear to involve two processes: the triggering of emergency response in the amygdala and the inability to activate the neocortical processes that generally balance the arousal (LeDoux, 1994). At these times emotion, unregulated by reason, swamps the system and the balanced integration of reason and emotion is lost. Thus certain stroke or brain-damaged patients, depending on which area of the brain is damaged, demonstrate either catastrophic fears or lack of impulse control, whereas others with lesions on the right hemisphere are unduly cheerful. The left prefrontal lobe appears to be part of the brain's "off" switch for disturbing emotions. It appears, then, that the amygdala arouses emotions and the prefrontal lobe douses them. The connection between the two is crucial for adaptive functioning. It is these connections that constitute some of the syntheses that serve as the basis of emotion schemes.

The development of awareness of feelings as well as improved self-regulation are important aspects of both the therapeutic process and treatment goals. The ability to be aware of feelings, regulate anxiety, and self-soothe are the crucial skills of life. Indeed, the inability to regulate anxiety is at the core of much dysfunction. Ultimately therapeutic change involves addressing dysfunctional emotion-regulating strategies and redeveloping more adaptive ones.

CHAPTER THREE

Emotion Assessment

ALTHOUGH EMOTIONS EVOLVED to enhance adaptation there are a number of ways in which this system can go wrong (Izard, 1979). All of us have experienced moments in which, against our best intentions, we hate our children, rage at those we are close to, fear authorities, envy our friends, feel intensely vulnerable with or jealous of our lovers, or feel disgust or anger at only the slightest provocation. When these emotional states are chronic, they stem from complex internal processes based on learning histories in which adaptive emotion expression and regulation has not been fully achieved. In dealing with emotion, we need to distinguish the particular nature of the emotion evoked. This requires assessing different emotional states and processes. In this chapter we will distinguish between various types of emotional processes. These distinctions will make it easier to understand emotional dysfunction discussed in the following chapter.

INTERIOR- AND EXTERIOR-RELATED EMOTION

In order to understand emotional experience, we must first make a fundamental distinction about the nature of the emotion. We need to determine whether it is related to the environment or the self. Some emotions give meaning to things in the world, offering information about them in relation to our well-being. For example, fear of the dark alerts us to the possibility that there could be something dangerous lurking there. Other emotions, however, are solely interior, referring to the self's experience. These emotions function to alter the self and its goals. For example, fear of the destructiveness of one's own anger leads to its suppression.

These two types of emotional reaction require distinctly different types of intervention. Reactions to the world need to be accessed for their information and adaptive action tendency and *expressed* in an appropriate manner. Self-referring emotions, on the other hand, need to be *explored* for their meaning and the nature of the internal relations that are generating them.

A client who comes into a therapist's office feeling angry at her boyfriend for forgetting their date is in quite a different state from that of another client who is angry at herself for failing to get there on time. In the first case the anger may be an adaptive response and its communication encouraged. In the latter case the client's anger at herself needs to be explored for what it says both about her standards and her violations of them. This exploration may lead either to an exploration of her overly harsh self-criticisms or to identifying a feeling of being overwhelmed, or even to some desire to not be on time. Expressive and exploratory interventions thus need to be tied to different types of emotional reaction.

OVERCONTROL AND UNDERREGULATION OF EMOTION

Clients may overcontrol or underregulate their emotions, and the goal is to help them with appropriate affect regulation. Thus the therapist needs early on to assess whether to work with a particular client to help access overcontrolled emotion or to help regulate undercontrolled emotions. Certain clients chronically deny their experience of feelings such as anger, sadness, or fear. They avoid emotion and need to learn to attend to experience and express feelings. Other clients whose predominant emotional responses are out of control need to learn arousal management, self-calming, and self-soothing strategies, as well as learning to attend to other more primary emotional experiences, such as hurt and fear.

There is a general consensus among clinicians that for certain psychological problems it is useful for clients to "get in touch with" their feelings. Certain problems stem from chronic avoidance or overcontrol of core affective experience. In pathological grief reactions, for example, the person has avoided the painful and normal emotions associated with profound loss and is unable to recover. There is a growing consensus that the blocking of important emotional experience in grief and posttraumatic stress disorder, for example, interferes with healthy functioning and prolongs rather than alleviates suffering (Horowitz, 1986; Herman, 1992; Pennebaker, 1990).

Moreover, the inability to access feelings and personal meanings, by being overly rational and intellectualizing in order to protect self esteem or avoid distress, is viewed as a characterological style that prevents effective coping. For example, a client with this style had been shamed and humiliated for any show of emotion and therefore had learned to disavow and distrust his emotional self. He was highly intellectual and overcontrolled, was unable to form intimate relationships, and said he felt like a shallow phony. Clients like this need to learn to attend to their feelings in order to accurately assess the impact of events on them and access their personal meanings. The inability to do this interferes with functioning.

In certain problems the inhibition of primary emotion can paradoxically result in problems of undercontrol or underregulation of related affects. This can be observed in people with poor anger control, where the problem is denial of underlying hurt or fear. Other people with unresolved primary anger toward a significant other can displace their anger onto others and are overly emotionally sensitive and reactive. Other instances where expression of affect is exaggerated, such as chronic alcoholic rage, depressive hopelessness, or hypervigilant anxiety, can also result from avoidance of more primary feelings of sadness, grief, or shame.

In a highly impulsive person with a fragile sense of self and unstable relationships, however, emotions often need to be regulated so as to prevent destructive expression and help calm the client. Thus underregulated rage, self-contempt, and shame need to be recognized as such and symbolized in words. This helps provide some distance and control, and slows down the overwhelm process. At this point self regulating strategies need to be learned. The client needs to develop ways of soothing him- or herself and providing self- comfort and self-support rather than panicking and acting impulsively or becoming overwhelmed by anxiety or shame.

TYPES OF EMOTION

In addition to the above overarching distinctions between exterior- and interior-related emotions, and over- or underregulation of emotion, a global three-part process-diagnostic scheme for assessing emotional experience and expression in therapy has been developed (Greenberg & Safran, 1984a, 1984b, 1987, 1989). Emotions according to this scheme can be seen as either primary, secondary, or instrumental. This is a functional scheme, one that distinguishes among diverse emotional processes that require different types of intervention.

An expanded version of the initial scheme is shown in Figure 3.1, and the type of intervention for each type of emotion is presented in Table 3.1. We trust that these classificatory schemes will become more differentiated and continue to grow as the skills of emotion assessment in therapy become more refined. These categories of emotion make

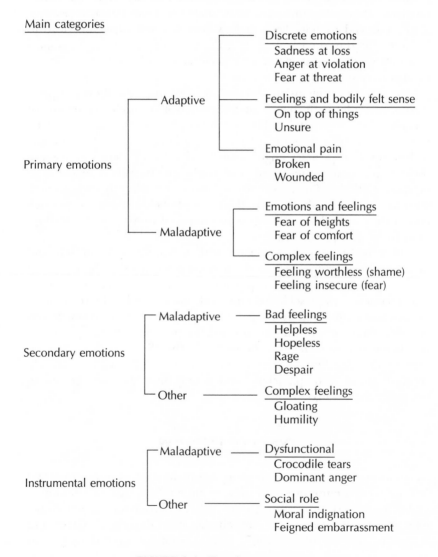

FIGURE 3.1. Emotion assessment.

clinically meaningful distinctions that guide intervention. As is indicated in Table 3.1, it is most appropriate to access primary adaptive emotions for their information, restructure primary maladaptive schemes, explore secondary bad feelings, and raise awareness of the function of instrumental emotions.

TABLE 3.1. Types of Intervention

Main type	Specific type	Intervention
Primary adaptive	Discrete emotions Sadness at loss Anger at violation Fear at threat	Access for adaptive information action tendency and need
	Feeling and bodily felt sense On top of things Unsure	Symbolize for meaning and need
	Emotional pain Broken Wounded	Allow and complete
Primary maladaptive	Emotions and feelings Fear of heights Fear of comfort	Access core maladaptive scheme for restructuring
	Complex feelings Feeling worthless (shame) Feeling insecure (fear)	
Secondary maladaptive	Bad feelings Helpless Hopeless Rage Despair	Attend to and explore
Secondary (other)	Complex feelings Gloating Humility	Awareness and exploration
Instrumental maladaptive	Dysfunctional Crocodile tears Dominant anger	Increase awareness of the interpersonal function and/or secondary gain
Instrumental (other)	Social role Moral indignation Feigned embarrassment	Awareness and exploration

Primary Emotions

In the scheme we first describe primary emotional responses, which are the fundamental, or initial, emotional response to external stimuli. These are distinguished from secondary and instrumental responses. The latter two types follow primary emotions and/or are more highly mediated and socially influenced. Each response in this scheme can also be seen as having adaptive and maladaptive subtypes. We first will discuss the subtypes of primary emotion that include (1) biologically adaptive and (2) learned maladaptive emotions.

Primary Adaptive Emotions

Primary adaptive emotions are fundamental states for which the adaptive value is clear—for example, sadness at loss, anger at violation, and fear at threat. It generally makes sense to protect one's territory from predators, attempt to reunite with a person who is missing, or run from danger. This category can be further broken into three subcategories: (1) *discrete emotions,* such as fear, anger, and sadness— these provide information and specific action tendencies; (2) *feelings*— these include a person's bodily *felt* sensations and the more complex felt sense of meaning or experience; and (3) *emotional pain*—this is a holistic system response providing information that trauma to the whole system is occurring.

Feeling and emotional pain do not have specific action tendencies but do provide adaptive information. When one is working with feeling it is the adaptive information and complex meaning that need to be symbolized. Pain, on the other hand, needs to be allowed, faced, and completed.

The discrete emotions are highly distinguishable patterns of response tendencies to stimuli. In therapy one often works to access such primary discrete emotions as sadness at loss and anger at violation. These emotions are attended to and expressed in therapy in order to access the adaptive information and action tendency to guide problem solving. They are core and irreducible responses and therefore are not explored to unpack their cognitive–affective components. For example, anger at maltreatment is a primary, irreducible, and core emotional response that needs to be evoked and symbolized in therapy in order to access the adaptive action tendency to push the offender away and establish appropriate boundaries.

We distinguish emotional pain from the basic, discrete emotions because pain appears to be a holistic system response to system fragmentation and trauma (Bolger, 1996). It also is adaptive because it informs us about hurt or injury that needs attention and needs to be avoided in the future. However, rather than being anticipatorily pro-tective, as are a number of the discrete emotions, it teaches people to avoid the pain-inducing situation in the future. Pain that needs to faced and completed will be discussed more fully later in this chapter.

In addition we distinguish feelings and a *bodily felt sense* of meaning (Gendlin, 1964), or complex feelings, from basic discrete emotion. Feelings most fundamentally involve physical sensations in the body but do not involve an action tendency. The term "feeling," used as a verb, encompasses the conscious experience of all affectively laden material; thus one feels an emotion, feels pain, or even feels a need. Feelings, in our view, encompass body sensations, such as warmth, tension and pulsations, as well as the more differentiated bodily felt sense referred to as "experiencing." This is a complex felt sense that results from the automatic synthesis of sensation with a variety of different levels of cognitive and affective information and produces integrative emotional meanings. This felt sense, when symbolized in awareness, produces a complex feeling that orients us in a complex interpersonal world and gives us our high-level "sense" of things such as feeling "on top of the world."

With regard to feeling it is interesting to note that as well as feeling specific sensations and more complex feelings, people are probably always feeling something more diffuse, in the times in between the more specific feelings. These background feelings are the brain's awareness of the person's ongoing body state, the disturbance or alteration of which is recognized as a change and as a more specific feeling (Damasio, 1994).

The discrete primary emotions result in expression and goal-di-rected action tendencies such as anger displays or flight. These affec-tive responses are innate and organized and depend on processes in the lower brain. The experience of these emotions, however, involves awareness of them, and they therefore are always to some degree synthesized with other levels of processing. Feeling an emotion thus involves experiencing body changes in relation to, and integrated with, the evoking object or situation and one's past emotional learning. Consciously feeling the emotion in connection with the object evoking it, rather than simply engaging in adaptive action, gives people more control over their reactions and allows them to learn from their own emotional reactions.

Feeling emotion allows for the formation of emotion associative networks or schemes, because consciously feeling something involves higher levels of the brain, and ultimately involves a synthesis of emotion, cognition, motivation, and action. Emotion schemes once formed then produce more complex bodily felt feelings when activated. These now no longer are a result of purely innate discrete responses but are a result of acquired responses learned under the influence of innate emotional responses.

In therapy, we want to access, unpack, and explore primary emotions. These are often complex emotional responses. What makes them primary is not simply that they are biologically based but that they are the person's *initial* or fundamental response to an event or experience. For example, a client who had experienced virtually no emotional support from a dominant, achievement-oriented father and a passive mother came to feel that having feelings and needs was not worthwhile because they were never responded to. He came to therapy with marital problems and feelings of emptiness and meaninglessness. Therapy worked toward helping him become more aware of his feelings and emotions, of present and past hurts, which lay behind his emptiness and bitterness toward his wife. He eventually contacted his deep sadness, his disappointment, and his present desire for nurturing from his wife. These primary, complex feelings did not simply reflect an innate, discrete, emotional response of sadness at loss, although they included it. Rather, they provided a consciously experienced sense of his sadness as influenced by his past learning about his sadness. Primary feelings are thus highly idiosyncratic, and subtly and uniquely customized to each individual. They act as crucial guides to which we often need to refer, to enhance reason and decision making.

Primary Maladaptive Emotions

These are primary emotional responses that have become dysfunctional, such as the fear associated with different types of phobias or fear of comfort or touch. These generally are based on learning and are embedded in emotion schemes. Other more complex maladaptive primary emotional responses include shame at self-expression or revelation, anger at others genuine caring or concern, joy at the suffering of self or others, and feelings of worthlessness or insecurity. These are generally based on pathogenic learning histories of extreme neglect, abuse, or invalidation that result in the formation of core maladaptive emotion schemes. The evocation of these schemes results in maladaptive *primary* responses to situations. They are primary because they are not reducible to any preceding or underlying emotional responses. These responses were generally initially adaptive, such as learning to fear closeness because it was associated with disappointment, control, or violence, or feeling shame because one's efforts or expressions were humiliated. Alternately, they are maladaptive responses of an over-stressed or dysfunctional complex system, as in panic, in which a variety of biological, biochemical, affective, cognitive, and behavioral factors combine in a manner to automatically produce a dysfunctional fear response (Barlow, 1985).

We have found that fear and shame are the primary maladaptive emotions that occur most often in our therapy. These primary maladaptive emotions are generally embedded in a weak, bad sense of self. These emotions need to be accessed in therapy, generally not for their adaptive response tendencies but in order for the core maladaptive emotion schemes in which they are embedded to be restructured by new in-therapy experience. The complex maladaptive self-schemes most prevalently associated with fear and shame are those of feeling either worthless or like a failure, the "bad me" sense, or feeling fundamentally insecure or anxious, the "weak me" sense.

For example, a client who had been harshly criticized as a child had felt hurt and rejected and had coped through anger and acting out. This behavior elicited further negative responses from others, and he felt powerless to change the situation. This eroded his confidence and self-esteem or sense of self, which remained weak when he became an adult. His weak/bad emotion scheme, when activated, led him to shrink away from social contact, to feel that people did not respect him and that they could see his lack of confidence. What was needed was to change the maladaptive emotion schemes that generated his sense of self and his complex bodily felt meanings that were associated with social contact. Maladaptive feelings such as these embody this man's unique experience of situation–emotional response relations from the past.

Secondary Emotions

These are the second broad class of emotions important for differential intervention. These emotions are reactions to identifiable, more primary, internal, emotional, or cognitive processes—thus secondary in time or sequence to internal processes. They can be secondary responses to primary emotional responses, such as expressing secondary anger when feeling primarily afraid as is sex-role stereotypical of men, or crying when primarily angry, as is sex-role stereotypical of women, or secondary responses to cognitive processes, such as feeling depressed when thinking about failure.

Secondary emotions can be subdivided into what we will term "bad feelings" and "complex feelings." Unlike primary emotions, both result from complex internal sequences of cognition and affect. According to our categorization, bad feelings include secondary reactions of hopelessness, helplessness, depression, and anxiety, as well as secondary rage, fear, and shame. Distinguishing these from primary adaptive emotion is important in therapy because intervention involves either bypassing or accessing and unpacking these secondary reactions to arrive at more primary and adaptive experience.

For example, a client who was trapped in an unhappy marriage with a controlling husband came to therapy expressing secondary reactions of sadness, depression, and a sense of hopelessness and resignation about how miserable she was. During therapy the client recalled having had an affair and described this as a time when she felt truly alive. This memory brought tears to her eyes. The therapist directed attention to her primary feelings with the response, "Sounds like there's a part of you that longs to feel like that again." The client in turn responded that it was "a crying shame" and talked about her regrets about all the wasted years with her husband. Through acknowledging the sadness of this loss, the client experienced her longing to be alive. As therapy progressed, the client became increasingly committed to connecting with the feeling part of herself, to not stifling herself, and to nurturing herself. The focus of therapy shifted from general awareness training to becoming more aware of her anger at her husband and identifying what she needed in this relationship. This helped her become more assertive in her marriage, and to be less willing to sacrifice herself for her marriage and for the sake of her family. Here secondary bad feelings of sadness, depressive hopelessness, and resignation were explored to get at the client's more primary feelings of sadness at loss of self and anger at being controlled.

Often, what is referred to as an emotion includes the person's reaction to the emotion and relationship with it. It includes the discomfort with, evaluation of, and inability to accept the emotion. When people feel unaccepting of or threatened by an emotion, they do not experience the emotion itself but rather the consequence of being unable to experience the emotion. People are often afraid of their anger, ashamed of their fear, and angry about their sadness. In these situations, what is referred to as an emotion, be it rage, jealous anger, or helplessness, is often a secondary response to the primary emotion. The response is an emotional reaction, often a defensive reaction to an emotion. Secondary feelings frequently are used to avoid some other more frightening, shameful, or painful feelings. Thus people feel anger to avoid sadness or fear to avoid anger. In contrast to primary emotions and basic human needs, this type of defensive emotion can be maladaptive and can lead to destructive behavior. Thus rage that hides grief, or acting out that deadens pain or hides a longing for care, is self-destructive rather than adaptive.

Similarly depression and anxiety can be complex secondary reactions to sadness, despair, loss, or threat, or even to depression and anxiety itself. Here people are depressed about being depressed, and fear their fear. For example, a client who had become depressed about the loss of her job chastised and hated herself for being depressed, believed she "should be over it already," and became more depressed, helpless, and immobilized by her inability to "get over it." These are all complex, self-reflexive processes of reacting to one's emotions and transforming one emotion into another. Crying, for example, is not always true grieving that leads to relief, but rather can be the crying of secondary helplessness or frustration that results in feeling worse. Clients who ask, "What is the point of bellyaching here when I do it all the time at home?" need to be taught the distinction between tears of helplessness, on the one hand, and therapeutic weeping (which could relieve helplessness) on the other. Emotions, especially when they are not symbolized in awareness, rapidly turn into other emotions: sadness, hurt, shame, or fear often turn into anger; fear turns into coolness; jealousy, into anger; and anger, into fear. This provides great complexity for client and therapist alike, and much therapy involves exploring secondary emotions in order to access more primary emotions.

In contrast with the secondary bad feelings above, some complex secondary feelings are not necessarily aversive or distressing. Feelings such as gloating or humility could be complex secondary feelings because they are secondary to a prior cognitive affective sequence. However, they are not necessarily experienced as bad feelings. In addition, any other emotion such as pride or joy or hope that comes after a more primary experience of, say, anger or after imagining a future event is a secondary feeling that is not maladaptive.

Instrumental Emotions

These are emotions experienced and expressed because the person has learned that they have an effect on others. They can be consciously intended in order to achieve an aim, or the person may have been learned without any awareness (i.e., through conditioning), that their expression has a specific effect and they have become habitual. Those that are consciously intended are constructed in order to influence others or to manage one's image so as to appear in a desired manner; those that are habitual are enacted automatically. From an early age children learn that emotional expression is very important in communication and they learn both in awareness and without awareness how to use emotional expression, and how to regulate it, in order to influence others. Thus people express anger in order to dominate others and sadness in order to evoke sympathy. These can often become chronic patterns of expressed helplessness and crying in order to be rescued, or anger and bullying in order to stave off taking responsibility. For example, a client realized that she expressed how depressed she felt whenever her husband expressed a need for support. Making this connection revealed that she often "showed" greater depression in order to get him to support her and keep him in the strong role. Another client realized that he expressed anger toward his parents to punish them and keep them at bay.

In therapy, maladaptive instrumental emotional reactions feel manipulative or superficial. They do not ring true and have the effect of distancing rather than touching the therapist. Therapists react to vocal quality such as high-pitched crying in the throat, rather than from the "gut," as indicating that clients are not deeply involved in their own experience. The therapeutic goal at these times is to help people become aware that their expressions are not necessarily helping them meet their needs. Appropriate interventions include helping people become aware of the instrumental nature of these experiences, and interpretations and exploration to understand the interpersonal function of the emotion and or the secondary gain.

In even more complex social constructions, people show certain emotions in order to be perceived in a certain way. Thus people, on being told of a moral or social transgression, may express dismay or moral indignation in order to impress others with their superior sensibilities, without necessarily feeling anything. Or people when inappropriately dressed for a social function, may express embarrassment in order to convey that they are well socialized and know the rules. These are all emotional responses constructed with differing degrees of awareness in order to achieve a social aim. People with high socioemotional "intelligence" are particularly skilled in this level of emotional expression.

Instrumental emotions are the emotions that social psychologists, social constructionists, and systems theorists think of as "roles" or "social constructions." Rather than "having" these emotions, people are regarded as "showing them" in order to achieve an effect or sometimes because the effect produces specific gains for them. They are considered communicative devices, and thus people are seen as showing anger and depression rather than being angry and depressed. They are also viewed as involving manipulation.

It is important to conclude this description of different types of emotional expression by saying that we are not claiming that primary emotions are real and the others are not real. All emotions feel, and are, real, in that they are experienced as feelings. All are experienced as a complex aspect of being. They do differ, however, in whether they are predominantly primary, secondary, or instrumental. The crucial clinical issue remains one of how to assess these emotions and distinguish among them in order to intervene appropriately.

HOW TO ASSESS EMOTIONAL STATES

Therapists use the following five sources of information to make ongoing assessments of clients' current states:

The first is empathic attunement to feelings involving the imaginative entry into the world of another and the tacit apprehension of a pattern of subsidiary information (Bohart & Greenberg, 1997). Thus, in listening to a client tell about his angry overreaction to some problems his son was having, the therapist sensed that the client also was struggling with feelings of not being able to live up to his own expectations of himself. Empathic attunement to these feelings of disappointment, in addition to his fears for his son, deepened his exploration significantly.

A second crucial source of information is nonverbal cues. We assess emotion from the analysis or observation of nonverbal expression, from attending to breathing, sighs, posture, vocal quality, and facial expression. Thus directing clients' attention to their curled lips of contempt or shallow breathing of fear will help them become more aware of their experience. In emotionally focused therapy (EFT) a sigh is worth a thousand words, and verbalizing what the sigh is expressing will lead much more directly to core experience.

Third, knowledge of universal human responses to prototypic situations provides a further source of information. Here the therapist's understanding as well as life and therapeutic experience is a factor. Cross-cultural responses can vary; knowledge of culture differences clearly helps her or him to understand how emotion is expressed.

Fourth, knowledge of a client's own emotional makeup and personal history provides a rich source of data that grows as the therapy progresses. The therapist comes to know over time that this client is prone to secondary anger when hurt or another client expresses fear when angry. Awareness and knowledge of our own emotional responses plays a critical role in knowing others. Personal therapy, experiential training, and awareness of one's own emotions thus are all important in enhancing the therapist's emotional awareness.

Finally, different types of personality styles and disorders also need to be taken into account in assessing emotion. The emotional expressions of people with different styles and disorders do not resemble each other in manner or meaning (Benjamin, 1993, 1996). For example, anger in people with borderline-type personality styles or disorders often occurs when the caregiver is seen as neglectful or abandoning. This anger is driven by panic and fear that the other doesn't care enough, and it is sometimes instrumentally expressed to force the caregiver to provide desperately needed attention. A person with a histrionic style may display instrumental anger to get praise and admiration; a person with an antisocial disorder expresses anger that is cold and designed to maintain control or distance. People with a narcissistic type of personality style often express secondary anger if their needs are not automatically met. Thus anger generated by panic, by a desire for admiration, by a need to gain control or take advantage of another, or from a failed sense of entitlement tends to occur more often in certain types of personalities. All require understanding of their function. Each represents a unique underlying core experience. EFT aims at accessing the core feelings and needs underlying all these different instrumental expressions of anger.

Finally, it is important to recognize that for some people, or for any person at particular times, attending to or evoking emotions of any kind may be unwise. When people are too fragile or too anxious, when there is too much cognitive disturbance, or when people are struggling to control overwhelming emotion, it can be harmful and damaging. In general, it is not profitable to evoke the emotional experience of psychotics and people with severe borderline personality disorders. When working with people with hysterical personality styles or in hysterical states, emotional expression of the emotion involved in the state should not be encouraged, although other emotions can be profitably accessed.

PAIN AND BAD FEELINGS

Two subtypes of emotional experience described above, emotional pain and bad feelings (which include both depression and anxiety), require special attention in emotion assessment. It is these experiences that so often bring people into therapy. Again, the distinction between pain and bad feelings is important in terms of how it influences intervention. Broadly, emotional pain is adaptive but frequently is avoided, and it is the chronic avoidance of pain that can be maladaptive. A common example of this is the inability to grieve over a major loss. Intervention therefore involves overcoming avoidance and accessing the painful experience. On the other hand, bad feelings such as depression are themselves maladaptive, and intervention entails accessing and changing the underlying cognitive and affective processes that generate the bad feeling state.

Painful Emotion

Pain is a bodily felt, primary emotional experience that, although adaptive, has only limited escape value. This is different from the more anticipatory primary emotions such as fear and anger, which are designed to promote action to prevent undesirable occurrences. Emotional pain is somewhat of a puzzle. It is not simply the experience of distress/sadness but is a complex feeling state. It is about both loss and damage—loss of relationship and damage to cherished aspects of self. People report that anger, sadness, and shame are all connected with pain. Intense emotional pain is experienced as anguish or agony, feelings of overwhelming suffering or distress. Pain is associated with the heart, often with having a broken heart, and is referred to as being deep and profound as well as explosive and overwhelming (Bolger, 1996). When feeling this kind of emotional pain, people feel out of control and experience physical pain in their bodies—in their heads and in their stomachs. They report feeling overwhelmed and fear being unable to stop crying, fear losing control. People report feeling weak, shattered, broken, ripped apart, having gaping wounds, and feeling empty and hopeless (Bolger, 1996). Pain, then, is a high-level sense of trauma to the whole self and is felt in a bodily manner as the "whole" self being broken or shattered. One client, experiencing for the first time the pain of never having had her mother's love, sobbed, "I have a big gaping hole inside. How does a person ever fill that up? I feel like she murdered me."

A client who had lost an infant had been unable to bear being present at her deathbed. Many years later, in therapy, she expressed the pain of this experience. Overcoming her fear of being shattered, she opened her protective shell and experienced the pain she had been attempting to stave off for years (Bolger, 1996). Rather than breaking, as she had feared, she found that she could access both internal and external support that would help her continue living with greater resolve. Having allowed her pain, she talked about all that her loss had meant to her and the way it had dramatically influenced her life.

Pain is not associated with an action tendency to prevent harm, but it does possess survival value. It achieves this by teaching one to avoid things that have been discovered to be harmful. Pain, as we have said, is not protectively anticipatory because it is experienced only after the damaging event has occurred. Although primary emotions, such as fear and anger, clearly alert us to impending dangers and threats and prepare us to meet them, pain tells us that something bad has happened and teaches us to avoid it happening again. Intense loss, violation, and denigration are threats to the self and cause intense psychological pain. People then attempt to escape facing such annihilating threats by cutting off their feelings and developing various other ways of avoiding these painful emotions. When pain becomes unbearable, people seize up and numb themselves, detach themselves, shut themselves off, and disconnect. Avoidance of pain and of the associated primary emotions is ego protective but, if chronic, is not adaptive because it cuts people off from their primary orientation and response system. Pain signals damage and a need for attention and repair.

Feeling the pain that has been avoided, although initially frightening and highly draining, often leads to relief, to feeling alive and connected again. It can lead to letting go and to a feeling of peace and tranquility. Clients often report feeling "exhausted but lighter, just good" or "drained but hopeful—hopeful that things can change." In therapy we always process the experience of allowing emotional pain and respond to the positive aspect, to the adaptive feeling of relief or release. Therapists need to ask clients how they feel after deeply experiencing emotional pain and recovering from it. Validating responses like "Exhausting, isn't it?," "Yes, it's hard work," and "Let go, just let the tiredness wash over you" are all helpful.

Children who grow up in abusive environments, or who have experienced other trauma and the associated primary emotions of fear and anger in a context of helplessness, learn to cope with the pain by automatically pushing away the distress or by unconscious dissociation. Certain aspects of experience or parts of self that "contain" the traumatic feelings, memories, and thoughts are blocked from awareness. The person feels numb to the experience or, in more extreme cases, may dissociate from it. In unstable and abusive environments, children learn that it is dangerous to be vulnerable and open about their feelings. They learn not to trust others, to avoid seeking comfort from others or relying on others. They suppress their own feelings and become increasingly unaware of them. They thus do not experience aspects of emotional life that are essential for normal development. In the absence of safety, support, and comfort, a sense of security and trust is not developed, and autonomy and independence can be impaired.

Painful awareness is split off or disowned in order to protect the self from feeling overwhelmed. Thus the rage, pain, and anguish of being abused is disassociated to protect the person from awareness of the reality of their situation. The person may feel afraid without knowing why or feel nothing at all. These unacknowledged experiences need to be reowned in therapy and worked through from an adult perspective. It is important also to realize that these parts of self-experience were adaptively split off at the time in order to protect the child from being overwhelmed. For example, a client who had been physically and verbally abused by her mother could recall feeling like a cowering animal hiding under a chair while her mother was poking and jabbing at her. She was aware of feeling afraid of being hurt but had never acknowledged the tremendous pain she felt that this was her mother, the person she relied on for love and protection. The realization that her mother wanted to hurt her was excruciating. This memory encapsulated fundamental operating assumptions about life such as "I am no good" and "Trust no one." She became tough and numb to the pain and lashed out first, before anyone else could hurt her.

Bad Feelings

Bad feelings, in contrast to emotional pain, result from something not functioning properly or smoothly within, from disharmony rather than from damage or trauma. Feelings that one is in conflict, guilty, worthless, anxious, or depressed are signals of internal problems, that there is something wrong that one needs to attend to. Secondary bad feelings are not purely adaptive signals about our reactions to situations. Rather, they are often signs of complex system dysfunction, of internal disorganization and disequilibrium, of hypersensitivity and reactivity to interpersonal threat or loss, and an inability to regulate these.

Bad feelings demand that we pay attention to what is happening internally in order to facilitate system reorganization toward greater equilibrium and internal harmony. For example, intervention with one client involved saying, "It sounds like a part of you is feeling sort of unsafe and weak, like you feel in some kind of danger that you can't protect yourself against in this new relationship." This is an invitation to explore the feeling of danger.

Although bad feelings in themselves are disruptive they still do provide a means of regulating the complex biological–psychological–social system that is the whole person. As we have said, the emotion system initially only had to deal with organism–environment interactions. However, with the development of the ability to reflect on ourselves, to represent, imagine, and consciously remember, emotions also become responses to our own processes. Emotions became responses to intraorganismic interactions as well as responses to the environment. Emotional "disorder" thus often reflects states of internal disorganization or hyperactivity that, if attended to, can be important precursors of reorganization.

Bad feelings that trouble people result not from primary emotional responses to environmental contingencies but from the evaluation and control of these primary responses. Much *enduring* bad feeling thus comes from attempts to control primary feelings that, if simply accepted, would themselves dissipate. In addition, bad feelings result from other forms of intrapsychic disharmony and dysfunctional processes, such as internal conflict, from complex cognitive affective sequences, from dysfunctional beliefs about oneself and one's world, and memories of unresolved situations.

For example, a client felt torn between wanting to end her marriage and fearing the consequent financial difficulties and disruption of the family. Intervention with this bad feeling entailed unpacking both sides of the struggle—the desires ("I want to be able to follow my own needs and feelings. Something has died between us.") and the fears or values ("the family is worth sacrificing oneself for—that's incredibly important to me . . ."). This exploration led to her understanding how she had sacrificed herself for her husband and to an awareness of her need to define herself more clearly. Another client felt angry at her parents for their lack of support, then guilty for not being a dutiful daughter, then tense, and finally powerless. She would give up and collapse into depression. Intervention entailed following the sequence of cognitive–affective processes producing the bad feeling, identifying the collapse into depression as it happened in the session, and accessing her unacknowledged primary response. The therapist responded, "You just suddenly collapsed, lost your power—somehow it's difficult to be angry at them. What happened to you just now . . . as you got close to your anger?" Similarly, with another client, who had been verbally abused by his father and unable to protect his mother from the father's beatings, the secondary bad feelings of depression came from his sense of himself as weak and bad and the world as unsafe. Intervention here entailed accessing and restructuring the complex maladaptive emotion scheme formed in childhood situations.

These examples demonstrate that bad feelings are the result of complex internal cognitive–affective sequences. They are generally secondary reactions to *underlying* more primary intrasystemic emotion processes or structures. Whereas primary feelings involve immediate and direct appraisal in relation to concerns and involve immediate reactions to situations, such as anger at violation and sadness at loss, bad feelings are more complex secondary responses. They are best understood as signals that something is wrong.

One common bad feeling that clients describe is that of feeling "upset." Feeling upset then is a general signal that something is amiss. The term upset connotes disorder, disarray, confusion, feeling disturbed, agitated, and stirred up. Upset generally occurs secondarily to primary anger, fear, and hurt. It tells us that some other emotion is attempting to break through. Often we feel upset without quite knowing why, without having registered the event, our construal of it, or our emotional response to it. All we are left with is the bad upset feeling. This bad feeling, then, is not the same as the primary feeling such as anger or hurt that elicits it. It is an awareness of irritability, say, which indicates that we need to search internally for what is troubling us. For example, a client recalled his first homosexual experience of being raped by an older boy and said he found it very upsetting to talk about this experience. The therapist responded, "Yes, I can imagine," but rather than making assumptions about the nature of the upset, further explored it by saying, "As you think about that now, what gets to you the most, what's the most troubling part of the memory?" The client responded that he was embarrassed, ashamed, and afraid that the therapist would find him disgusting. The therapist told him that this was not so and further empathically conjectured, "somehow something is disgusting about that experience. . . ?" The client went on to talk about his shame at having found it exciting, his self-doubt that maybe he "asked for it," anger at the perpetrator for "making me gay," and hatred of his own sexuality. In this case, exploring the surface-level upset feeling accessed more primary emotional experience as well as core pathogenic beliefs.

Two Sources of Bad Feelings

Bad feelings appear to result predominantly from either *intrapsychic* processes, such as disowning, self-control, and self-evaluation, or *interpersonal* processes involving hypersensitivity to dependence and control, and overconcern about loss of connection and loss of autonomy.

Bad feelings that occur in response to intrapsychic experience result from negative evaluations of experience, attempts to control primary feelings, internal conflict, and self-criticism. In addition, bad feelings result from maladaptive internal cognitive–affective sequences that lead to intensification of negative feelings. The bad feelings associated with lack of self-acceptance, for example, involves self-castigation and self-denigration for experiencing feelings that are construed as unacceptable. Thus a person may feel guilty or contemptuous toward the self for feeling afraid or for feeling angry or envious, or a person may feel anxious and upset about wanting to be close but being afraid to assert this need. In the foregoing example of a client feeling self-hatred about his homosexuality, subsequent interventions would heighten awareness of his specific self-criticisms about his sexuality and the experiential effect this self-castigation has on his sense of self. He would experience the bad feeling of rejecting a part of himself.

The second major source of bad feeling is the emotional response to interpersonal ruptures predominately associated with perceived rejection or criticism. These are the ruptures of an emotional attachment bond and the bad feelings related to issues of interdependence. One of the important functions of emotions is to inform us that a relational bond is at risk—that we are in danger of losing it or that it is becoming threatening or violating. The primary emotional responses to relational ruptures are anger, sadness, or fear, and these responses are basically adaptive. It is only when, for a variety of reasons, these cannot be properly regulated that we begin to get secondary bad feelings. Such secondary reactions include feeling overly dependent, angry, or depressively withdrawn when our needs are not met, feeling afraid of closeness or separation, and feeling distrustful or sensitive to disapproval. Loss of connection with, or disapproval by, others is upsetting and can cause depression and anxiety, as can fear of intimacy or fear of loss of interpersonal control. Interpersonally generated bad feelings are most intense when the other person is a significant attachment figure. Sequences of despair, anger, and depression result from separation and abandonment.

For example, a client's marriage was characterized by long periods in which her husband would ignore her. She would feel intolerably lonely and would go through the following cognitive–affective–behavioral sequence. She first would desperately try to engage him, to reconnect. When he still did not respond, she would fly into a rage. This would be followed by self-castigation for her outburst and a sense of futility and hopelessness, feeling that things would never change. She then would collapse into depression, with a weak/bad sense of self. Another client who had been strictly controlled by her mother while growing up had learned that relationships were constraining. She found herself feeling panicky and claustrophobic in current relationships whenever intimacy demands were made of her. She felt unable to maintain her own boundaries, feared losing her sense of herself, and wanted to run. Here, getting too close was experienced as a boundary intrusion and produced fears of engulfment or invalidation and left her deeply anxious. Therapy needed to help her use her anxiety signal as information that she needed to take control rather than feel controlled, and to relax rather than tighten up.

Bad feelings of this type are generally produced by complex cognitive–affective sequences and by difficulty in regulating feelings adaptively. This poor ability to regulate and self-soothe results in escalating internal sequences and finally *hyperarousal, hypersensitivities, and overreactions* to slights, rejections, or intrusions. These processes are generally based on a negative learning history. Thus a more dependent person, that is, one who has a high need for connection with others, reacts to mild rejection or distance with fear. If the fear is combined with attributions of blame and/or catastrophizing and memories of loss, the initial fear is intensified and transformed into panic and anger at being violated. For one client rejection was accompanied by the memory of her father saying to her when she was child, "You're an ugly little thing. Who would want you anyway?" The memory would cause her to fly into a rage.

Chronic and intense bad feelings associated with momentary ruptures in connections or minor conflicts with others stem from an inability to autonomously regulate the self's emotionality by self-soothing. It is important to teach clients these skills, either explicitly or implicitly, in therapy. The metaphor of the "inner child," although a cliché, can help people to access self-soothing responses. In the above example of the client who was deeply wounded by her father's denigration, the therapist said, "That's so hurtful! What would you like to say to support that little girl, what does she need?" This helped the client to say what the wounded child needed to hear. It was important that she soothe herself while the memory and the pain were still alive so that she could experience her need and the soothing words would spontaneously emerge from that need and so she could experience the calming effects of her own actions. Together they also discussed how this self-caring could be implemented outside of therapy and what kinds of self-nurturing and -soothing behaviors the client might engage in.

ASSESSMENT AND FORMULATION

We generally emphasize process-oriented, moment-by-moment forms of assessment and diagnosis, rather than an initial case formulation or behavioral form of assessment (Greenberg, 1991; Goldman & Greenberg, 1996, 1997). One defining feature of EFT is this ongoing assessment of the client's current cognitive–affective problem state. This includes an assessment of what type of processing and what type of emotional experience is occurring and what type it would be helpful to heighten or evoke at any given moment, and what type of emotional experience is to be bypassed, managed, dampened, or perhaps confronted. For example, a therapist might bypass secondary anger, which she or he recognizes by its content and manner of expression, and be attuned to the hurt indicated by a sudden breaking in the voice, or a shakiness in the angry blaming, that suggest some unresolved hurt and sadness at being ignored and feeling unwanted.

Clients also frequently experience more than one type of cognitive–affective processing problem. Victims of childhood abuse, for example, can experience both underregulation of emotion, in the form of impulsive anger, and overcontrol of pain and sadness. Process diagnostic assessment, therefore, pertains to assessment of a particular process, at a particular time, rather than to the client's global personality (Greenberg et al., 1993). Process diagnosis of current experiential states is central to working with emotion. It is the client's presently felt experience that indicates what the difficulty is and whether the problematic processes are currently accessible and amenable to intervention.

In the following chapter we will discuss sources of emotional disorder.

CHAPTER FOUR

Sources of Emotional Disorder

*T*O FACILITATE DIFFERENTIAL intervention it is useful to categorize emotional disorder into five broad potential sources of dysfunction: (1) the inability to effect changes in the relationship with the environment that are prompted by an emotion's action tendency, which results in stress; (2) avoiding or disowning of emotion, which leads to disorientation and incongruence; (3) problems in the regulation of emotional intensity, which lead to poor coping; (4) trauma, which results in a host of difficulties, often described as posttraumatic stress; and (5) dysfunctional meaning construction processes, which result in maladaptive emotional responses. Each one of these sources of disorder will lead to different types of treatment including stress management, facing avoidances, development of coping skills to improve regulation, emotional reprocessing to assimilate trauma, and restructuring of the emotion schemes generating meaning.

A further source of emotional disorder involves dysfunctional biochemical processes. Given that our interest in this book is in psychotherapeutic means of treating emotion, we will not concern ourselves here with purely biochemical sources and their treatment but will instead focus on dysfunction that results from psychological sources.

STRESS

The first major problem for the emotional organism occurs when the emotion does not achieve its adaptive aim of changing the relationship with the environment. When this happens the provoking stimulus remains and continues to evoke the feeling. Too much ongoing feeling, especially intense negative feeling, produces stress and eventual breakdown. Thus, if one continually feels afraid or angry but is unable to escape or define one's boundaries, the body becomes overtaxed and eventually breaks down. In these situations recognition and removal of the source of stress is therapeutic, for example, changes in lifestyle, changes in relationships, or changes in the work environment. Thus, when clients are in abusive relationships or failing at school, coping with the immediate situation takes precedence over more internal exploration.

AVOIDANCE AND DISOWNING OF EMOTION

If the evoking source is internal rather than an environmental event, the person may be placed in a situation comparable to the one described above. The emotional action tendency cannot achieve its adaptive aim of changing the organism–environment relationship because the person cannot leave the field. However, this time the field is within. When the self is not allowed to be transformed by the emotion, the person copes by attempting to prevent or avoid the feeling process by ignoring, denying, or distorting experience. People find many ingenious ways to avoid feeling their emotions and the pain associated with their emotions. However, for healthy functioning, such avoidances need to be overcome and new ways of coping implemented. When painful feelings are attended to and accepted, the pain can be endured and can be utilized as information that the system has been damaged, is in disequilibrium, or is disorganized and that something needs to be done to change the self and/or the situation.

Painful feelings by their nature are difficult to endure, and therefore people attempt to avoid them or interrupt their experience of them. For example, a client grew up with an extremely violent father. As a child, he feared for his own safety and powerlessly witnessed his mother being severely beaten. He learned to cope by numbing himself to his feelings of fear and rage and also learned to distrust any emotional displays. As an adult he was affectively flat. He had been unable to form a close relationship with his own sons, lacked energy in his work, and had not shed a tear over his mother's death. Intervention involved explicitly teaching him to attend to his internal experience, particularly his bodily experience. Thus, he was encouraged to attend to the tension in his stomach and to the rising sadness in his chest, and to exaggerate bodily signs, such as tapping his hand in agitation, in order to intensify his experience. One difficulty in working with clients like this is that emotional flatness permeates the session and the therapist struggles to find a spark of energy. However, in this case the therapist remained present-centered and explored the client's experience of flatness: "Even though you know you felt angry, now as you speak about that incident it's like there's a type of heavy blanket, a fog or cloud around your experience, (C: Yeah.) deadening it somehow, no energy in it. Can you go into that experience, really taste it, tell me about it, what it's like for you? Where in your body do you feel it?"

Another major source of dysfunction is estrangement from feelings whereby what people think they feel is not what they actually feel. For example, people can feel angry but think they should be forgiving, or feel sad but put on a happy social face. Their experience is not integrated. Internal signals are mixed. The angry or sad bodily experience is accompanied by tension, sometimes butterflies of anxiety, and they can become confused and collapse into helplessness. Intervention entails attending to bodily cues and unpacking and clarifying components of experience. The faster people are able to learn to be open to and accept their feelings, the sooner they are able to benefit from the information contained within them and the better they are able to cope with the world and their emotions.

Different types of information-processing strategies are used to control emotional reactions. These can result in the removal of the affective aspects of experience from awareness or in behavior that prevents the feeling from being experienced. Some people withdraw from or avoid situations that evoke disturbing emotion. Others ignore or do not acknowledge what they are feeling. They use distraction strategies such as humming or busyness, or transform their feelings into psychosomatic complaints. For example, people avoid disturbing emotions by not remembering the painful affective reactions associated with major life events, thereby not realizing the full impact of what occurred. This is evident in therapy with clients with externalizing styles who give detailed stories of events that leave the listener untouched. Others engage in stimulus-seeking or impulsive behavior in order to blot out their feelings. Extreme numbing behaviors such as self-mutilation, binge eating, drug and alcohol abuse, excessive masturbation, and promiscuity can be engaged in to dissociate from the painful feelings or to self-soothe. Thus impulsive behaviors have the same basic goal as overcontrol—to avoid feelings.

Feelings enhance our capacity to cope and, once accepted, can better be coped with themselves. Their avoidance, on the other hand, leaves us doubly deficient. First, the adaptive information is neglected, leaving us disoriented. Second, the avoidance fails to make the feelings and their effects disappear. Rather, it leaves us incongruent, with our feelings, thoughts, and actions in disharmony. Our physiology and sensorimotor system are in one state, our words and conscious thoughts are in another, while our intermediate experiencing process is caught between the two. This impedes our ability to cope, to act on our emotions effectively, for we are unable to assert our boundaries or seek comfort. People who chronically avoid feelings no longer automatically attend to the felt referents of their experience, do not symbolize emotions in awareness, and are unable to create new felt meanings and promote action relevant to their well-being. Once feeling is blocked, people are unable to carry forward their experience to the next step. Rather, they remain stuck in a state of continued avoidance.

For example, a client came into therapy to deal with troubling feelings toward his estranged father. He had successfully suppressed these feelings until his father suddenly reappeared in his life. The client valued ideas of serenity, meditation, and emotional control, yet he felt confused, happy, sad, and angry. Exploring his anger toward his father in therapy was very threatening, and he began having anxiety attacks. Therapy entailed, first, mutual agreement that overcontrol or avoidance of emotion (particularly anger) was part of the problem and that collaboration was needed on the goal of overcoming avoidance at a pace he could tolerate. Exploration of his anger was balanced with teaching skills for managing his panic attacks. Second, therapy focused on exploring the avoidance process as it occurred in the session. The therapist helped him become aware of how he avoided emotion, often by blanking out whenever he felt angry, and helped him identify the physiological and cognitive strategies he used to suppress his anger. By attending to his presently felt experience, he became aware of how he stopped breathing for a moment and deflected his attention to a spot on the rug when anger threatened. His fears and beliefs about anger— that it leads to loss of control and to loss of connection—were accessed and explored. The experiential consequences of his avoidance were explored, such as alienation and ultimately anxiety when feelings threatened to emerge, and slowly he became more able to tolerate his anger and his grief without fearing they would annihilate him.

PROBLEMS IN REGULATION

At times it is the regulating process influencing the dynamics and quality of emotional experience that is itself problematic. The intensity, lability, quickness, duration, recovery rate, and persistence of our emotions can sometimes be the source of maladaptiveness.

It is thus not simply the generation of the anger or the hurt that is maladaptive, but it is the person's inability to regulate the dynamics, the intensity, or duration of the hurt or anger that is the problem. Anger becomes rage, hurt becomes devastation, and anxiety becomes panic. For example, in the aforementioned client who became panicky when he felt his anger toward his father, the issue was to help him regulate his anxiety about being angry. The therapist thus helped him to learn to regulate his breathing, to soothe himself with reassuring statements like "It's OK, go slow, take your time," and to understand his panic as anxiety about his anger.

Although regulation of intensity is important in life, this is not to suggest that intensity of experience and expression is always maladaptive. It also provides color and passion to life. All of us, however well modulated, sometimes adaptively lose our cool, and this is to be expected at certain times and in certain people.

Emotions are also subject to regulating action in a variety of different ways. It is not only a matter of modulating intensity. Events, for example, can be sought out or avoided in order to regulate emotional experience. Responses based on emotional memory also need to be regulated; otherwise, past experience could overly govern present responses. Moreover, automatic emotional reactions can be regulated by secondary appraisals of coping abilities and by planning how to cope with experience. Emotional experience can also be modified by selective attention and reattribution. In addition, the action tendency can be checked or changed and the felt impulse or urge can be suppressed so as to disappear from awareness. Distress can be regulated by self-soothing, fear by self-calming (whistling in the dark), and anger by counting to 10. Thus emotions can be managed. Emotion regulation develops over a lifetime, and much of it involves a synthesis of emotional responses and learning and at the brain level a coordination of the emotional response and higher-level reflective processing. Regulation is not always conscious or voluntary; in fact, most regulatory processes are not in immediate awareness.

Two automatic processes, excitation of an action tendency and its regulation, are thus involved in the production of one emotional response. It is the synthesis and balance of these that result in the final emotional expression and experience. When regulation fails, excitation can escalate and become dysfunctional. This is exemplified in the case of a client who had a history of being battered in his family and who experienced unresolved anger about being sexually abused in his childhood. When he began to think about that abuse he would become incredibly angry and would lash out at anyone who crossed his path. Intervention with him did not entail heightening his emotional arousal, as his anger was already aroused and often displaced onto others. Rather, the therapist helped him manage his arousal through attending to (regulation of) breathing and helping him soothe himself and focus on the appropriate target of his anger. An emotionally focused treatment needed to help him appropriately express and resolve his legitimate primary anger at sexual violation in childhood, which had had devastating consequences for his self-esteem and sexuality. Thus, rather than becoming overwhelmed with rage, he learned to breath while simultaneously verbally expressing his anger at the batterer, articulating the effects of the violation on him and holding the batterer accountable for the harm. All this occurred while he received support and validation from his therapist. Therapy also needed to help the client go beyond the anger to access and experience other disowned aspects of the emotional experiences associated with the abuse, such as his feelings of powerlessness, hurt, and sadness. Finally, emotionally focused therapy (EFT) enabled him to soothe himself, while feeling all these painful emotions, again with the help of an empathic supportive therapist.

The regulation process can be dysfunctional both in terms of under- and overcontrol of emotional experience and expression. There is clearly often a need to modulate some type of emotional expressions while dealing with problems caused by overregulating them. The regulation process can also be seen as sometimes being dysfunctionally involved in enhancing, augmenting, or creating an emotional response. One can get madder and madder by dwelling on a grievance or can intensify crying in order to ensure sympathy. Impression management and falseness can involve processes of appearing to feel.

As well as regulating the intensity of primary emotions, regulation also involves the management of complex secondary affective responses such as depression, anxiety, and frustration. Here regulation involves not becoming overwhelmed or debilitated by bad and confusing feelings. To not be taken over by a depression, to not collapse at a setback, or to not panic when one is scared are important coping skills. Difficulty in regulating bad feelings and painful emotions are central to many of the problems of people suffering from affective and borderline personality disorders. Much of the intense emotional experience and expression involved in these disorders is either secondary to more primary feelings or is instrumental, involving a learned use of emotion in order to achieve an interpersonal aim. Regulation of these feelings then involves slowing down highly rapid escalating internal reactions. It involves reducing the intolerable rages or the scathing self-contempt and being able to contact the more modulated primary feelings that are lost in the rapidity of the unfolding of the internal sequence.

In addition to regulating the *expression* of emotion, the development of the *experience* of basic security in the self is in our view one of the fundamental tasks of affect regulation. For many individuals, developing capacities for affective self-regulation in areas of distress is at the heart of the change process. To be able to regulate anxiety and affective arousal by developing the ability to calm fears helps a person to feel safe and secure and to maintain a sense of self-coherence and competence. The failure to develop this ability results in much disruptive emotionality.

In therapy it is often the soothing presence of the therapist that is important to help people acquire the ability to soothe themselves at times of great distress. The therapist's ability to be empathically attuned to a person's affective state and to genuinely accept and value their experience helps clients develop the capacity to become self-empathic and thereby contain their own experience. In addition, in therapy the slowing down and reorganizing of cognitive–affective sequences helps clients deal with many runaway secondary emotions, while the ability to put feelings into words and to bring reflective awareness of consequences of expression to bear on aroused emotion helps in their regulation.

TRAUMATIC EMOTIONAL MEMORY

Trauma is a significant source of emotional disorder. It shatters people's sense of reality and leaves them with emotional memories that continue to plague and overwhelm them (Herman, 1992; Janoff-Bulman, 1992). Posttraumatic stress disorder results from a dysfunction in the emotional response system.

Trauma that results in extreme emotional arousal leaves people with highly terrifying, vivid moments stamped in memory. Posttraumatic stress results from intense reliving of these experiences. The memories are often intense perceptual experiences in which the sight, sounds, and smells, the sight of blood, the shriek of another victim, the smell of gunfire or of an abuser's alcoholic breath, or the feel of his unshaved stubble are experienced in the present again. These symptoms are signs of the activation of the emotional brain and of it forcing these memories to intrude into awareness. These intrusive memories are triggered by the slightest cues and are a major symptom of emotional trauma.

The emotional brain acts as a fast-response system, and when this is integrated appropriately with neocortical regulation it acts as an adaptive response system. The emotion alarm system can, however, be inappropriately triggered as a result of unresolved trauma. This system can become dysfunctional when it produces alarm signals that do not fit the situation. There appears to be a special memory process for highly emotionally charged experiences that have especially aroused us. Such moments of high arousal appear to be imprinted in emotional memory with special potency. The emotional memory system in addition can operate independently of the neocortex such that emotional reactions and emotional memories are formed without conscious mediation. The amygdala can thus house emotion memories and response repertoires that were formed under conditions of high arousal without conscious awareness and, when activated, produce experience and actions without us quite knowing why we feel or act the way we do.

This memory system initially provided an evolutionary adaptive advantage ensuring that we would have vivid memories of intense emotional experiences and automatic reactions to them. It can, however, become dysfunctional as a result of trauma because the rapid-appraisal system searches for elements associated with these past memories and can activate a response before full confirmation occurs that the match is correct. This produces an intense response in the present, similar to that which occurred in the original high-arousal or traumatic incident of long ago. But now this response is to a new situation only vaguely similar to the past situation, and this results in dysfunctional responding.

In addition to adult traumas such as violence or terrorization that leave potent memory imprints, many powerful emotional memories of childhood abuse date from early years, when symbolic and narrative capacities were not fully developed. This leaves a person with potent emotional learned repertoires that are difficult to understand because they are stored in emotional memory in an unsymbolized manner. They result in emotional responses unaccompanied by words to help in their comprehension of them.

It is often the uncontrollability in the traumatic or catastrophic experience that makes that experience emotionally overwhelming. The feeling of helplessness seems critical in inducing subsequent posttraumatic stress, and the fearfulness can be accounted for by changes in the limbic system (Charney, Deutsch, Krystal, Southwick, & David, 1993). Changes appear to occur both in brain circuits and in the hormones related to emergency fight or flight responses. These act to alert the body to emergencies that are not there in reality. Although these responses are adaptive in an emergency, when the brain changes because of trauma such that a person is always in a heightened state of readiness to respond to even minor cues with alarm, the person becomes highly vulnerable.

When such traumatic memories become embedded in brain functioning they interfere with adaptation, the normal learning process, and with relearning that it is safe and that more normal responses to minor threats are adaptive. In treatment the fear or intense emotional reaction may need to be aroused to some degree to be reprocessed in the safety of the therapy situation. The traumatic experience needs to be symbolized and put into narrative form and integrated with the experience and recognition that it is now safe. By putting the sensory material in emotional memory into words, the memories are brought more under neocortical control and can be integrated into a person's meaning structures (Van derKock, 1996). Reliving the experience in therapy with the safety and security of an empathic, supportive therapist provides the person with a new experience. Experiencing the high arousal occurring in tandem with the therapeutic safety, the client begins to relearn that the terror can and does subside and that he or she is truly safe. In children traumatic situations are often reenacted, or worked with in play therapy, in order to symbolize and restory the experience and to reempower the child. In addition to symbolizing experience, people who have suffered trauma also need to learn to calm themselves. This occurs in a variety of ways. First, they need to understand that their symptoms of hyperactivity, hypervigilance, and panic are symptoms of posttraumatic stress disorder and not signs that they are losing their minds. Second, they need to learn to regulate their physiological arousal. Finally, they need to learn to combat the helplessness by gaining a sense of control in their lives (Herman, 1992).

DYSFUNCTIONAL MEANING CONSTRUCTION

Another major source of emotional disorder is based on faulty meaning construction. In our view emotion dysfunction is not primarily a function of conscious dysfunctional or irrational thinking. Rather, it results from problems in the complex cognitive–affective structures and processes that automatically generate subjective meaning and emotional experience. Problematic core experience, such as feeling worthless or insecure, arise from core maladaptive emotion schemes. These complex structures synthesize a variety of levels of information processing to generate personal meanings. Moreover, dysfunctional secondary emotions, such as hopelessness and rage, can occur as a function of complex, learned cognitive–affective sequences.

The Error of Assuming Cognitive Error

Early cognitive therapists hypothesized that it is verbally mediated faulty appraisals, automatic thoughts, and erroneous thinking and beliefs that are the cause of emotional disorder (Beck, 1976; Ellis, 1962). In our view these cognitions are more a result of tacit emotional processing than a cause of it. Dysfunctional emotional meaning construction does not generally arise simply from *errors in thinking or faulty appraisals* of reality. Thus, for example, when one is approaching an attractive person, it is not necessarily an irrational thought or faulty conscious appraisal that rejection is likely (when no evidence of rejection is there) that is the source of dysfunctional fear of rejection. Dysfunction results rather from tacitly synthesized emotional meanings.

While it is true that conscious thinking or verbally mediated reasoning can and do lead to feelings and that erroneous thinking can lead to dysfunctional emotional responses, it does not mean that all emotion and all problematic emotions result from thinking conscious or automatic thoughts. There is no doubt that consciously reflecting on personal circumstances, changing a decision, or altering a way of thinking clearly can change your feeling. Thinking about an exam you have failed or thinking that you have been poorly treated by others can and does generally result in feeling bad. Automatic thoughts and the cognition–emotion link, the proposed major source of dysfunction, and the target of change of much cognitive therapy (Beck, 1976; Ellis, 1962), although involved in the production of secondary bad feelings, are in our view not one of the major causes of disorder. Rather, we propose that automatic thoughts are produced by the conceptual system and are involved in the maintenance of emotional disorder. Any linear sequence hypothesis, such as thinking leads to feeling or vice versa, however, is far too simple. Rather, multilevels of processing of sensory, propositional, and imaginal information, as well as complex mutual interactions of thinking and feeling, must be taken into account (Greenberg & Safran, 1987). Ultimately, however, it is emotionally toned subjective meaning that comes from the experiential processing system, not thinking from the conceptual system, that is of critical importance in meaning construction.

Bad feeling, as one can check against one's own experience, results far more from the implicit meaning involved in the rupturing of interpersonal connectedness and from the evocation of emotionally laden perceptual images and scenes in the mind's eye than from explicit, linguistically formulated, specific negative thoughts. The latter rather result from an initial emotional orientation or sense of the situation. Feeling is at first a nonlinguistic representation to oneself of one's bodily state.

This has implications for EFT. There are many situations in which people conceptually "know" that their thinking is irrational or illogical and still cannot stop or control their reactions. Interventions then need to be aimed at accessing and unpacking the emotion network or meaning structure generating their reactions. Such exploration focuses on bodily felt emotional experience in the session and this internal focus, in the context of a safe and supportive therapeutic relationship, allows for the admission of new information that modifies the associative network.

One's experience of reality is constructed from the synthesis of perceptual, sensorimotor, motivational, and memorial information as much as from conceptual linguistically formulated thoughts. It is the thoughtless image, the wordless automatic sensorimotor response, and the felt meaning of the look or touch of another or of the sound of her or his voice that often governs emotional responses, rather than an explicit thought. Unmediated by conscious thought, these emotions and feelings influence subsequent thought and action. It is thus our clients' emotional sense of themselves in their world and their emotional reactions to events that needs to be evoked in therapy and exposed to new information if we hope to reorganize their construction of meaning and modify their bad feelings.

Overemphasis on Beliefs

In our view, semantic beliefs about oneself or one's world also often are the result, rather than the cause, of dysfunctional cognitive–affective processes or bad feelings. They too result from complex meaning construction processes. Beliefs such as "I won't survive if you are distant" or "I am worthless if I do not succeed" do not operate in *conscious awareness* to determine bad feelings and related action. These beliefs are themselves the result of complex constructive processes. Bad feelings are generated by complex expectancies about goal attainment, constructed from past experience. The experiential system's appraisal of the probability of attainment of one's needs, goals, and concerns is at the heart of an emotion scheme. When these schemes are activated and their outputs are synthesized into consciousness, they produce responses of panic and desperation *as if* a belief such as "I won't survive if I'm rejected" or "If I fail I am worthless" is operating. Although it is therapeutically helpful for people to become aware of their response patterns and to symbolize them in propositional form, articulating the type of belief that appears to govern their reactions and experience, it is not necessarily always the case that the conceptual belief actually preexisted and led to the response. More importantly, rational disputation of these beliefs will not result in a change in the emotional response. Rather, it is the enduring expectancies about goal attainment, based on schematically encoded regularities, that need to be changed. These are changed by new experience, not simply by reasoning (Greenberg & Safran, 1987; Safran & Greenberg, 1991).

EFT then evokes the encoding structures and opens them to new experience rather than rationally disputes beliefs. Articulation of experiential regularities, as verbal beliefs, is helpful because it gives a person greater awareness and a sense of control. Examples of change by new experience, as opposed to by reasoning, are seen repeatedly in work with clients who have been sexually abused and feel guilty. Even though they may now intellectually know that as children they were innocent and that they were coerced, and this is somewhat helpful, they still feel worthless or bad. In EFT the empathic responses that validate shame and embarrassment—such as "It's hard to talk about" or "Some sense that you must have asked for it, even though you know this is ridiculous"—are far more helpful than pointing out the irrationality of these feelings. These clients need, in therapy, to reexperience the abusive situation with the support of the therapist, in order to access alternate experience of themselves in their gut, as truly feeling violated and being truly innocent. This is a deeper "knowing" than reasoning alone.

It is a deeper knowing than conscious belief or thought that produces felt meaning and experience. It is the sensorimotor and bodily felt feelings, generated by the multilevel emotion schemes and their complex syntheses, that *result* in the negative thinking rather than vice versa. It is these emotion schemes and the bodily felt sense that are the primary therapeutic targets in EFT. These are accessed by focusing on what is felt, or by attending to how one feels as one is saying something, rather than focusing only on what is being said. This involves attending to a bodily felt sense rather than a thought.

What Produces Dysfunctional Meaning and Feelings

Emotion schemes are the complex meaning construction structures that produce dysfunction. These are based on evaluations of the complex patterned characteristics of a situation in relation to the individual's need/goal/concern. Emotional meaning is the product of the complex interaction of many elements, The need, goal, or concern guiding the individual, in the particular situation, is however a central element in the meaning the situation has for him or her. Thus feelings of anxiety and threat of rejection, in approaching a member of the opposite sex, arise only to the degree that one approaches the other under the goal of seeking a romantic connection. The appraisals involved are not thoughts but rather automatic evaluations along fundamental survival-oriented dimensions, such as goal relevance, uncertainty, danger, novelty, or pleasure (Frijda, 1986; Scherer, 1984). These dimensions are tacitly evaluated and initial personal meaning arises not from thinking but from rapid automatic appraisal of match/mismatch between the situation and the need, goal, or concern a person brings to the situation. Conscious thinking and more complex meanings are generated subsequent to the initial emotional processing in order to elaborate personal meanings. EFT clinicians thus are attuned to and respond to emotions and core need/goal/concerns implicitly or explicitly expressed. This elicits exploration of meaning.

In our view passion has really never been successfully ruled by reason. Moral imperatives or reasoned argument only succeed in changing emotions where they themselves become emotional. There is no doubt that in therapy one hopes ultimately to help clients' change negative thinking. However we view conscious cognition more as the dependent variable and believe that changes in emotional structures will lead to a change in thinking. Our approach to therapy is therefore designed to change thinking by changing the *emotional* experience and affective goals that lead people to think in dysfunctional ways.

In simple terms, when people feel angry they think angry thoughts, when they feel sad they think sad thoughts. For example, obsessive thoughts and compulsive behavior are generated by an underlying state of insecurity, and it is the complex sense of insecurity that needs to be addressed. The obsessive thoughts are by-products of this fundamental insecurity. Alternately it is fairly common for people who are feeling depressed to find themselves thinking, "I wish I was dead." Although these thoughts are operative to maintain the emotional states, they did not necessarily cause them and challenging the thoughts will not alter the emotional state. Rather, the emotion schemes involving the needs/goal/concerns evoked by the situation and the evaluation of whether or not they will be met generate emotional meaning. It is this emotional meaning construction process that needs therapeutic attention.

A crucial aspect of therapeutic change then involves identifying the person's primary emotional responses and the goals that govern this processing. Once the need/goals/concerns have been identified, they facilitate new self-organizations based on a new sense of goal directedness or on the letting go of needs/goals that cannot be met. For example, a depressed and anxious client who was typically overly self-sufficient says, "Yeah, I just want to curl up and make the world go away. I want to have someone take care of me, do it for me." Although this may sound depressive, it actually is an important step in the change process. By acknowledging her feelings of wanting support, she is letting go of her need to be radically independent and "do it all herself." Now she can begin to open herself to support, first from the therapist and later from others.

The Depression-Producing Meaning Construction Process

The depression-producing process depicted in Figure 4.1 further concretizes the functioning of the emotion schematic meaning construction process. Although it is not possible to truly capture depressive functioning in a flow diagram, this figure incorporates several fundamental observations. First, in many instances change in depression by noncognitive means leads to change in negative thoughts (Simons, Garfield, & Murphy, 1984). Second, depressive mood clearly leads to negative thoughts and state-dependent memories (Clark & Teasdale, 1982). Third, in many situations it is impossible to identify negative automatic thoughts preceding bad moods, and in many clinical instances changes in negative thoughts do not lead to change in feeling. Fourth, on different occasions the same negative thought can have very different effects, sometimes producing bad feelings and sometimes having little or no effect, implying that it is not the thought itself but the vulnerability to it, in the form of activation of a weak/bad sense of self, that seems important (Greenberg, Elliott, & Foerster, 1991; Paivio & Greenberg, 1995).

In Figure 4.1 we see that in response to an event, often a major life stress, the person's apprehension of loss or failure generates an emotion of, say, sadness/distress. This emotion, with its attendant tendency to withdraw, is the primary emotional response. In a dysfunctional depressogenic response, a weak/bad sense of self (a maladaptive emotion scheme based on a history of loss or damage), fear and shame, and automatic thoughts then are activated by the sadness/distress. The initial emotional reaction evokes a schematic prototype of this emotional experience that is stored in memory. In depressive experience the negative thoughts are activated by the emotion scheme itself, by the primary emotion response, and by conscious conceptual processing. Thus when people feel sad or blue

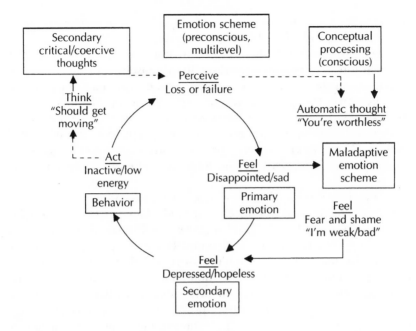

FIGURE 4.1. The depressive process. *Note:* Emotion is a process that unfolds dynamically over time without a definite starting point. We apprehend the personal meaning before we consciously appraise a situation (checks for novelty, pleasantness, personal significance). Different kinds of cognition enter into various stages of the emotional response. The body (sensations, feelings, moods, passions) contributes to subjective experience, a process that goes hand in hand with appraisal. Thinking does not have a controlling executive role, as indicated by broken lines.

they often think depressive thoughts. It is important to note that in our view it is the activation of the *core maladaptive emotion scheme* by the primary emotion that is central to the production of both a lasting set of negative cognitions and a weak/bad sense of self characteristic of depression. Thus feeling sad or distressed in response to a loss or failure "pulls for" or evokes the depressive weak/bad sense of self formed from the person's life experience. Recently Smith (1996) demonstrated that depressed subjects showed an elevated proportion of negative emotion memories of the more distant past. This indicated that their memories were not so much about the recent life stress that precipitated the depression but more about some earlier life experience. This finding supports the idea that it is the evocation of a core maladaptive emotion scheme that is important in producing depressive experience.

Negative thoughts themselves are not the sole target of EFT intervention because negative thoughts themselves are not essential in producing the primary feeling state or the weak/bad sense of self. The negative thoughts rather are important in maintaining the depressive state. In addition, negative thoughts that arise purely from conceptual processing are ineffective in producing enduring bad feelings. They simply "bounce off" a secure or competent sense of oneself rather than activate the weak/bad emotion schematic processing.

Thus it is the initial sadness/distress that activates a maladaptive emotion scheme and produces fear and shame and an enduring weak/bad sense of self. This negative self-scheme is the person's preexisting vulnerability to depression. Learned negative cognitions, such as the self-evaluation "You're worthless," depicted in Figure 4.1 acting in conjunction with the emotion-evoked core scheme, exacerbate and maintain the depression. The activation of negative thoughts and of the weak/bad sense of self then produces the secondary emotional response of hopelessness and the enduring depression. Again, notice that the depressed hopeless feeling is more directly linked to the emotional memories connected with primary sadness and disappointment, and to the associated weak/bad self scheme, than it is to the negative thoughts per se. All these elements are synthesized into the complex depressed bad feeling, the experience of hopelessness, and the resulting lethargy and inactivity. The process of depression also involves a second level of reflexive self-evaluation that the self is bad for being depressed, and this results in "coaching" the self more and more coercively and disparagingly to "snap out of it." This, in turn, produces further experience of failure or unworthiness, which further evokes emotion schemes related to failure and loss.

Problematic Factors in Meaning Construction

Emotional problems thus result from different problematic aspects of meaning construction, and each of these requires a different interventive emphasis. Problems in meaning construction arise from the following factors:

1. The activation of *dysfunctional meaning construction based on needs/goals.* Here the dysfunctional emotional meaning is based on the appraisal that certain *needs and affective goals* in a situation will not be

met. Intervention involves restructuring either the appraisal of mis-match or the goal governing the situation.

    2. A person's *dysfunctional reactions* to accurate automatic or conscious appraisals that needs will not be met. Thus a person who needs to be esteemed may overreact with rage to an appraisal of being slighted. Here the response to frustration or disappointment becomes the focus of treatment.

    3. *Negative evaluations of the self and of primary feelings or desires.* Here dysfunction stems from peoples inability to accept their own experience and it is the negative evaluations which are focused on therapeutically.

    4. Problematic *sequences* of feelings, thoughts, evaluations, and attributions in interactions. Here exploration of the sequences leads to greater awareness of primary experience and tacit meanings governing experience.

    These four complex processes, rather than faulty thinking, strongly influence subjective meaning constructions, bad feelings, and personal reactions. They are described more fully below.

Dysfunctional Meaning Construction Based on Need

The emotional meaning of a situation lies in its relevance to our needs/goals/concerns. The affective goal therefore organizes the situation and is important in the creation of meaning (Lewin, 1935). It is the evoked schematic complex, rather than the appraisal of a situation alone, that results in emotion. Thus highly distrustful clients often have high needs for control in relationships and the therapy situation itself. These needs come from prior experiences of being damaged or out of control and were motivated adaptive responses to their life experience. This frequently occurs with clients who have a history of childhood abuse. Appraisal of the current situation as controlling in conjunction with the need or goal to be in charge, or the fear of not being in charge, are all the focus of EFT intervention.

    In our view, the goals toward which cognition strive are ultimately set by affect (Pascual-Leone, 1991; Greenberg et al., 1993). Thus it is the affective goals (the need/goal/concern) that the person brings to the situation that are crucial in meaning construction and in dysfunc-tion. For instance, when an emotion scheme based on a need to be loved or liked is evoked, it organizes the situation in terms of accep-tance/rejection. Then, through the automatic apprehension of a pat-tern of cues, the person may begin to feel rejected. This apprehension is not a specific thought such as "I am unlovable" or "I am being rejected," but rather a bodily sensed feeling of being ignored or just hurt, based on tacit pattern recognition. It is this felt sense that directs cognition to analyze the situation for further meaning. It is only at this point that the conscious appraisal of rejection emerges, with its attendant thoughts and fears of being unlovable.

Again, an emotional response is not based on tacit appraisal alone but on this appraisal in relation to a need. If a need to be loved or accepted is not operating, an appraisal of rejection will not result in an emotion. Note that it is some form of scheme accessibility that is important here. If a particular emotion scheme is for some reason highly accessible or currently operating, it determines the current operating need/goal that structures perception of the situation for appraisal. For example, a depressed client often reacted to her boyfriend's nonresponsiveness as if it were abandonment, support, and security. In therapy this led to dealing with her unfinished business with her father, not changing an irrational appraisal.

In general, it is the affectively determined needs and goals brought to a situation that require therapeutic attention more than the appraisals they motivate. Thus in the treatment of hypersensitivity to rejection, as in the above example, it is an awareness of the need to be nurtured or respected and attendant fears, as well as the ability to act in order to meet the need, or tolerate its frustration, or relinquish the need/goal, that must be developed.

In addition to the distress caused by lack of awareness of needs/goals/concerns, much distress is produced by the inability to let go of unattainable needs/goals/concerns. This inability leads to repeated futile attempts to overcome discrepancies between appraised situations and desired goals. Thus the inability to let go or change one's goals can produce persistent attempts to reprocess information, replay the situation and redo it in one's mind. Clients remind themselves of the qualities of a lost person or experience in efforts to regain that lost goal or person. Therapeutic change often requires giving up emotionally based internal efforts to achieve the unattainable goal. This occurs by relinquishing or changing the goal, grieving, and *accepting* the loss or the failure (Greenberg, 1995).

Dysfunctional emotional meaning, then, is the result of a complex meaning construction process in which the organization of emotional meaning is based most fundamentally on people's current adult needs, goals, and concerns. Both the degree to which the emotion schemes are activated and the degree to which needs are judged as being satisfied determine distress.

Dysfunctional Responses to Mismatch

Highly important in dysfunction are the responses to a perceived mismatch between the person's need/goal/concern and the situation. Once again it is not simply a faulty appraisal that is problematic. Rather, there is a dysfunctional response to an accurate appraisal of mismatch—an appraisal that his or her needs will not be met. It is the sense of desperation about the concern or need not being met, plus the internal response sequence to this desperation, that results in problematic experience and behavior. In these situations we disagree that dysfunction then results from faulty primary appraisals. We also do not believe that dysfunction stems from a developmental delay resulting in infantile needs, as held by classical psychodynamic theory. Rather, dysfunction results from maladaptive *responses* to accurately perceived mismatches between situations and needs (i.e., to perceived need frustration).

Another common scenario occurs when one correctly perceives a situation but overreacts. In interpersonal hypersensitivity, for example, it is not a faulty appraisal of rejection or coldness by the other that is problematic. The appraisal may well be correct. What is problematic is the intensity or desperation of the emotional response to frustration of the need. It is one's feeling that, in response to distance, it is impossible to survive without the desired support or closeness. For example, the client mentioned earlier who felt abandoned when her boyfriend was not optimally responsive would then fly into a rage at his lack of caring. Rather than say she felt lonely, she would attack him. This intense reactions to the thought that needs will not be met can be produced by prior deprivation, learning, and/or complex reactions to disappointment.

To take another example, if you struggle with feelings of inadequacy, you may accurately appraise that you've come up short. The problem arises from the intensity of the response, which might have been more moderated at another time when you were feeling stronger.

For example, a client who was not accepted into graduate school fell into a profound depression and felt that she could not go on. Therapy validated her profound disappointment and teased out the meaning of the disappointment in terms of its damage to her core sense of self. It became clear that her reaction was based on her emotional sense that if she failed she was unlovable. In her childhood the only ways she had received her father's love was by excelling, and now she felt like no man would value her, thus her desperation. Even though she had "failed" to get into graduate school, the intensity of her grief came from other sources—loss and her unresolved feelings toward her father.

Self-Evaluation and Interpretation

Humans appraise reality in relation to needs and secondarily appraise or evaluate their own desires and emotional responses to the environment. Evaluations that anger, sexuality, or fear are bad will result in bad feelings. This form of reflexive self-evaluation and self-interpretation is constitutive of people's increasingly complex emotional experience of themselves. Thus it is people's relationship to their feelings that is important. This involves moral judgments that get their strong emotional meaning from a learning history in which chastisement produced bad feelings.

The evaluative process is always at work in the reflexive process of meaning construction (Watson & Rennie, 1994; Watson & Greenberg, 1995). In order for us to become conscious of experience, complex meaning has to be articulated, and this involves continual, progressive attempts to form what is initially inchoate into language. We put words to feelings and in so doing create conscious experience (Greenberg & Pascual-Leone, 1995). The articulation process shapes our sense of self and what we want, value, and believe. Self-interpretation and articulation thereby is importantly constitutive of emotional experience. Thus a construction of an implicit felt sense as feeling tired is quite different to a construction of it as feeling disappointed. Meaning construction and self-evaluation and the associated emotions generated by these complex processes can always be more or less adaptive. Therapy thus involves a process of attempting to symbolize experience in as differentiated and nuanced a manner as possible in order to capture subtle felt meanings.

Although articulating experience in language often helps constitute experience and certain forms of articulation help us view ourselves and the world differently, again it is important to note that these articulated propositions or thoughts did not preexist or cause our experience. Rather, it is the more complex automatic functioning of the rapid action emotion schematic system that produces emotional responses for symbolization in language (Greenberg et al., 1993).

Internal and External Sequences

As we have said, maladaptive responses of rage, anger, tearfulness, worry, or anxiety can be complex, mediated secondary reactions generated by cognitive–affective sequences based on past experience, learning, and present formulation. These sequences, and far more complex sequences, need to be unpacked and understood in therapy.

For example, the man discussed early in this chapter who had the extremely violent father, recalling the unfair physical punishment, exhibits a sequence in which he says he can almost feel the pain of his blows, then feels angry, then disappointed, then shuts down, and then becomes self-conscious, aware of the audio-recorder. Intervention then involves an exploration of his conscious beliefs, injunctions, inhibitions, and anxieties concerning anger expression. This client's belief system and self-esteem centered around self-control, which to him was inconsistent with anger. The experience of anger was highly threatening because it reminded him of his father and everything he did not want to be. It is this client's chain of responses to his own anger that are problematic and prevent the primary anger and probably sadness from being dealt with.

Complex emotional meanings also result from our ongoing evaluations of our own emotional responses in real time and from conscious construction of the meaning of situations as they unfold. Again, it is not a simple matter of appraising but rather a complex, highly context-dependent ongoing process or sequence that is at work. In dealing with dysfunction, then, it is the ongoing sequence of internal processes and of the attributions in ongoing interactions that need to be dealt with.

CONCLUSION

Emotions are responses that arise when situations are appraised as relevant to concerns. Emotions then can be viewed as our concern-satisfaction system (Frijda, 1986). The appraisals of the situation's relevance to concerns are neither rational nor irrational; rather, they simply ascertain whether there is a match or mismatch between the situation and concern. Affective goals or concerns are thus the final reference point in understanding the occurrence of emotions, and it is our response to these concerns being activated or goals not being met that requires therapeutic attention far more than do faulty appraisals.

PART TWO

INTERVENTION FRAMEWORK

CHAPTER FIVE

The Process of Change

*E*MOTIONALLY FOCUSED THERAPY (EFT) focuses on evoking automatic emotional reactions that are both adaptive and maladaptive. The safety of therapy and the increased effort of therapeutic work helps clients concentrate and focus their attention on internal experience. Under the increased attentional allocation to internal experience made possible by therapy, more information becomes available. This promotes attention to new elements of experience, particularly to alternate feelings and needs. Maladaptive emotion schemes, in their activated state, are exposed to new alternatives generated by focusing attention on emerging experience that arises in this altered state of awareness. Change of maladaptive schemes in therapy occurs, then, by the evocation of maladaptive emotional experience and the assimilation into it of newly accessed adaptive experience. This process of increased awareness and emotional accessibility helps create new schematic models of self-in-the-world.

IMPORTANT ASPECTS OF WORKING WITH EMOTIONS

Purely expressive or cathartic views of emotional change that use metaphors of "getting rid of" one's feelings or "getting them out" miss the mutative aspect of emotional experiencing in therapy. A number of crucial aspects of change-producing work with emotion are outlined below:

First, therapeutic work with feeling is a *stage* process. Acknowledging and expressing feeling is only the first step and is often insufficient, in itself, to produce enduring change.

Second, provision of safety and support is a crucial first stage. Much bad feeling involves feeling disempowered or a loss of connection. Therapists need first to validate clients' experience and help them to restore control of their feelings. Some aspect of control is regained when people are able to name and symbolize the experience and have it understood and accepted by another. No further therapeutic work can possibly be done until the client feels safe and able to control or master her or his own experience. Allowing painful experience includes the element of choosing to allow such bad or painful feelings rather than being overwhelmed by them and feeling out of control. A collaborative alliance to feel or reexperience is crucial in the process. If this does not exist, the client will appropriately resist going into these bad feelings. Once some sense of mastery exists and the person is not too afraid of these bad or painful feelings, has some sense of internal resources or skills for coping with them, plus the external support of the therapist, then it is therapeutic to go into the feelings. Premature reexperiencing of traumatic and painful feelings, without establishing a therapeutic alliance and clients' sense of control to help them feel protected, is tantamount to retraumatizing patients. This is to be avoided at all cost. Although it is important to encourage people, when ready, to face the dreaded experience, when in doubt it is better to err on the side of caution.

Third, in dealing with bad feelings as opposed to painful primary emotion, it is not experiencing of the bad feelings themselves that is primarily therapeutic. Clearly feeling hopeless or worthless is not itself therapeutic. Rather, secondary bad feelings *signal* that something is awry and experiencing them helps access what evokes them so they can be dealt with better. At times the secondary bad feelings signal the interruption of more fundamental emotion, such as when the onset of anxiety and panic attacks signals that long-suppressed anger and disappointment at an abusive father are surfacing. Then it is accessing these primary feelings that is important.

Fourth, often it is overcoming avoidance and interruption of feelings that is important. Attempting to prevent feelings is a method of coping with emotions that results in dysfunction. Overcontrol is mistaken for regulation, and too much attentional energy goes into avoidance and interruption. Rather than simply allowing emotion, it is often awareness and mastery of the avoidance or interruption processes that are crucial in lasting character change. Awareness and mastery of avoidance enable one to experience feelings when one so chooses and to keep feelings at a distance when one so desires.

Fifth, once the primary feeling, such as hurt at feeling unloved or anger at feeling violated, is accepted, it needs to be experienced and expressed but *also clearly symbolized in awareness* (Gendlin, 1962, 1974). In addition, its process of generation, causes, and effects need to be experienced in awareness. Symbolization of the "what" of experience, for instance, feeling insecure, plus awareness of the "how" of the emotional experience, as in how one's internal process leads to this, are often much more important in producing change than understanding the "why." Thus statements such as "I feel hurt because ..." often lead to conceptual explorations of immediate or early causes that take clients away from their presently felt experience.

Sixth, and of crucial importance, in addition to feeling the bad feeling and awareness of its generating processes, it is *accessing alternate emotionally based needs/goals and other internal resources* that helps one cope that makes experiencing such feelings therapeutic. Acknowledging and experiencing a bad feeling rather than getting rid of it leads to accessing other emotions and needs/goals and to complex cognitive–affective changes in which one's view of oneself and the world is changed. Once people access their adaptive emotions and strivings they begin to transform their rotten, powerless, unloved feelings into feelings of being more worthy, agentic, or acceptable. They become more agentic and begin to develop a future orientation. Now they are able to set goals and make plans, rather than ruminate on the past.

EMOTION SCHEMES AND THE SELF IN CHANGE

The role of emotional meaning structures in generating emotional experience is central in understanding emotionally focused intervention and is therefore described below.

For heuristic purposes we envisage a sequence (see Figure 5.1) in which a stimulus (S) is processed through a variety of levels of information processing of which the highest level is a complex mediating cognitive–affective structure or emotion scheme (ES). As stated previously, there are two distinct levels of meaning creation: the emotion-schematic, experiential level, and the conscious, conceptual level (CP). It is the former that is responsible for immediate emotion experience. The emotion-schematic level of processing leads to an experienced emotion response (ER) and possibly to some conscious thought (CT) or cognitive construal. Conscious thoughts, however, are influenced most directly by other levels of cognitive processing, particularly by conceptual processing (CP). The feelings and thoughts produced by these levels of processing mutually interact, influencing each other to produce emotional–cognitive (E-C) sequences and a

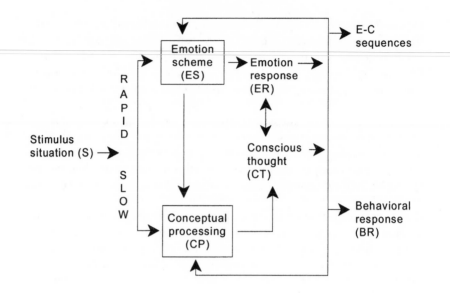

FIGURE 5.1. Emotion schemes in the construction process.

behavioral response (BR). All the components feedback and influence emotion scheme activation. EFT intervention deals directly with ER in order to attend to any adaptive information in it and to access the generating emotion scheme. Once the emotion scheme is accessed, differential intervention occurs, depending on the nature of the emotion scheme and its relation to the person's problem. If the scheme is maladaptive, it—and the processing that leads to its synthesis—becomes the target of treatment with the goal of creating alternative schemes. If it is functional, the experience that results is used to guide adaptation and problem solving.

We realize that personal realities are constructed in a much more multidetermined manner than is depicted in the mostly linear model shown in Figure 5.1 and that construction of meaning results from a dynamic synthesis of many elements and involves the person as an active agent (Greenberg et al., 1993, Greenberg & Pascual-Leone, 1995; Pascual-Leone, 1990a, 1990b, 1991, 1992). The sequence depicted in Figure 5.1 is a simple tool for understanding the role of emotion schemes in generating experience and in contrasting emotionally focused intervention to other forms of intervention.

Thus, EFT intervention can be contrasted with behaviorally focused interventions that aim directly at the BR, attempting to modify responses or change them by acquiring new skills and altering contingencies. EFT similarly can be contrasted with cognitively focused interventions that deal directly with consciously available and linguistically symbolized beliefs or thoughts (CTs), attempting to rationally refute them or collect evidence to contradict them. EFT also differs from the more conceptually oriented aspects of dynamic intervention that focus on insight into links across situations or distant causes of experience. Rather, EFT attends directly to, and explores in depth, the ER and the E-C sequences in a particular situation to access core emotion schemes and new change-producing experience. Thus, when someone is feeling bad, for instance, guilty or worthless, and articulates this as "I am too selfish" or "I'm a failure," it is the feeling state generating these thoughts that is focused on. Attending to the bad feeling leads to an exploration of the humiliation, the dread, or unacceptable wishes associated with and generating these views. By means of this focused exploration, the cognitive affective meaning construction sequences are unpacked until new core emotional experiences are accessed. New experience in these cases might be, in the case of selfishness, a true sense of entitlement to one's wish for happiness even at the cost of pain for self and others or, in the case of failure, a felt sense of one's worth in other areas of life. Access to new experience produces change in the activated ES and/or the processing that lead to their synthesis. Change in these schemes is thus produced by making previously inaccessible internal experience available to them in order to construct new schemes.

There are two major sources of this new internal experience. First, needs/goals/concerns and the internal resources to meet them, based on the primary adaptive emotional response system, are accessed (Greenberg et al., 1993; Perls, 1969; Perls, Hefferline, & Goodman, 1951). For example, when a client feels anxious and alone, accessing her sadness and her need for contact/comfort along with the attendant action tendencies are sources of new experience. Second, new interpersonal experience with a therapist, especially feeling that a fragile sense of oneself is heard, received, validated, and accepted, is a source of new transformative experience.

Accessing new goals, the first source, comes about largely by attentional reallocation. Here attention is directed toward new material and to needs/goals as they emerge in the session. Awareness and symbolization of emotional goals produces system reorganization and the utilization of new resources to meet the needs/goals. For example, a client who had been physically abused as a child, at a critical moment in therapy shifted her attention from her initial enduring fear-based goal of "slinking away like a dog," learned in the original

situation, to her newly accessed anger-based goal of boundary assertion. Another client, who had been desperately trying to make his
volatile marriage work, continually began each session with a litany
of complaints about how impossible his wife was. He entered one
session having just been hit by his wife and having had his efforts to
get away restrained by her. He began again to rail against her. The
therapist noted how angry he was and how he began every session
this way, but how hurt and powerless he must feel. He immediately
broke into tears. The therapist asked what he needed and he said,
"Peace and quiet and some safety." In response to the question "How
can you get this?" he said, "By leaving." Thus, he reorganized the
long-standing needs/goals to succeed in his marriage and to not
abandon his wife. This change of goals facilitated a new approach,
and he explored how his efforts to preserve the dysfunctional marriage had kept him locked in. He changed his goal from one of
succeeding at marriage to one of survival and peace, and this
crystallized a new course of action. He left the session with the
resolve to leave the house and returned the following week having
moved out, and with plans to end the marriage.

   New interpersonal experience, the second source of change, comes
from contact with a therapist who is being genuinely caring, empathic,
validating, and respectful, and is a source of new genuine interactions
that are emotionally corrective (Greenberg et al., 1993; Rogers, 1957).
For example, the client mentioned earlier who had learned to slink
away like a dog came to feel accepted by the therapist rather than
humiliated when she felt weepy. In another example, a client mentioned
in an earlier chapter who began having panic attacks after accessing
his suppressed anger toward his father, for the first time became angry
at his therapist and the therapy for having created his anxiety. The
therapist acknowledged and nondefensively validated his anger and
discomfort and the role she had played in its generation, and then
collaborated on better ways to manage his anxiety in the session and
at home. The client had a new experience of having his anger accepted,
taken seriously, and responded to, leading to constructive action rather
than rejection or the destruction of a relationship.

THE PROCESS OF CHANGE WITH DIFFERENT TYPES OF FEELINGS

The process by which change takes place with different types of
emotion are outlined below. First, the role of primary adaptive emotion
in change is discussed. This is followed by a discussion of changing bad

feelings. Embedded in this is a discussion of changing both secondary bad feelings and primary maladaptive feelings. Finally the transformation of pain is discussed.

Primary Adaptive Emotions in Change

Therapeutic work with primary adaptive emotions is the most simple and direct form of emotion work. The primary adaptive feeling needs to be accessed, acknowledged, and symbolized. The adaptive action tendency, mobilized by the emotion, as well as the need are symbolized to provide orientation and inform problem solving. Again, anger organizes people to set boundaries, fear organizes escape, and sadness organizes recuperative withdrawal, seeking of the lost object, or comfort.

Important therapeutic processes involve attending to feeling and bodily sensations, and symbolizing these in awareness. The point here is that emotion cannot serve its biologically adaptive function in a complex human environment if emotionally toned experience is not attended to and symbolized with accuracy and immediacy. This enhances orientation and aids problem solving.

For example, a client with pervasive boundary difficulties in relationships and an inability to express anger would collapse into depression and tears whenever she felt angry. Gradual emotional awareness training around her experiences of anger (feeling the energy in her body, standing or sitting up straight with her feet planted firmly on the floor, looking her imagined mother in the eye) helped her acknowledge and reown these feelings. A turning point occurred in therapy when she expressed her primary anger toward her mother for the beatings and criticism she had received—"I understand her limitations but I'm furious at her for what she did to me"—saying assertively that "She had no right to be so violent with me," "I didn't deserve such harsh treatment, I deserved better," "I needed support and encouragement, not this constant criticism," and "I refuse to accept her criticism and verbal abuse anymore."

In the case of another client, acknowledging primary sadness at being rejected by her husband was important. It was very helpful for her to say how much it hurt, how she didn't want to let go, how she felt like there was a big hole inside, and that she was afraid that the emptiness would never be filled up. Acknowledging the feeling was the first step in a process of mobilizing alternate resources to cope with her difficulty.

Another client sobbed deeply about her lack of mothering, the lack of love or caring in her life, and her deep need for this. This acknowledgement led to collaboration with the therapist to overcome this chronic pain and was a motivator in helping her look for other relationships to provide the nurturing and support she needed.

The Process of Changing Bad Feelings

Intervention with bad feelings, such as feeling hopeless, helpless, worthless, or vulnerable, is different from intervention with primary adaptive emotions such as anger, sadness, or fear in which the goal is to acknowledge the primary feeling for the information it provides and to access the action tendency. In addition, working with bad feelings does not involve a simple allowing, reowning, and reprocessing of experience as does working with pain. Bad feelings, rather, are a product either of primary maladaptive emotion schemes or of secondary emotions and complex cognitive/emotional sequences, and require a more complex set of interventions. There is no adaptive action tendency associated with feeling useless, worthless, helpless, or humiliated or with feeling chronic shame, or with feeling constantly rejected, nor does one live these bad feelings through to completion. Rather, bad feelings need either to be restructured or regulated. These processes are described next.

Accessing and Restructuring

Intervention with bad feelings always involves three phases. First, the secondary bad feelings such as hopelessness and vulnerability are evoked in the session in order to make the processes that generate these feelings accessible. Second, maladaptive emotion schemes, such as core feelings of insecurity and worthlessness involved in the generation of these bad feelings, are activated and restructured. Finally, new primary feelings or internal resources such as disgust, anger, *and* sadness and a sense of entitlement to care and support or needs for competence and mastery are contacted to provide an alternative to the core maladaptive schemes.

In dealing therapeutically with bad feelings more is needed than simple awareness and acceptance of what is felt. Emotionally and experientially oriented therapies in the past have not clearly articulated or communicated how people deal with bad feelings, other than appealing to the growth tendency. Partly this is because they have not distinguished between primary emotions, pain, and bad feelings.

Again, just getting in touch with secondary bad feelings is not, in and of itself, helpful. What is required is to enter into these states with sufficient resources to be able to cope with them in a new way. Working with bad feelings involves both allowing and acceptance of the feeling and a process of change in which something new emerges.

For example, a client who had been abandoned by her mother at an early age and then reconnected with her, kept looking to her mother to "prove that she loves me." The mother continually disappointed her by being neglectful and inconsiderate. The client felt victimized and powerless, and would collapse into depression and tears. While acknowledging her pain and hurt, the therapist pinpointed moments in which the client experienced resentment and indignation at her mother's behavior. The therapist then directed her attention to these and intensified them to help her access her anger and empower herself. In this case, collapsing into tears of powerlessness was not adaptive. Along with accessing anger and the new assertive, standing-up-for-oneself action tendency, her tears of powerlessness also were differentiated into more adaptive, primary sadness at loss. The latter was expressed, and led her to facing the reality of her mother's neglect and to letting go of her unmet needs for her mother's unattainable love.

A Model for Working with Bad Feelings

Based on our intensive analysis of audio- and videotapes of in-therapy situations in which clients experienced and worked through secondary bad feelings in EFT it appears that the performance sequence shown in Figure 5.2 is the one associated with change. First, the bad feelings, say, of feeling helpless or lonely and alienated, are aroused in the session. Once the feelings have been evoked, the client must attend to the feelings rather than avoid them. Next, the complex internal

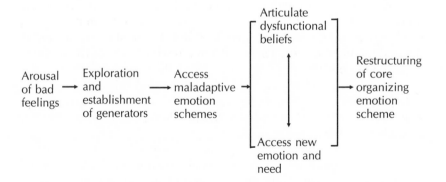

FIGURE 5.2. Restructuring of bad feelings.

processes producing the bad feelings need to be unpacked, differentiated, and explored in order to identify the dysfunctional cognitive–affective sequences that generate the bad feelings. Alternately, this results
in accessing a core maladaptive emotion scheme such as feeling
insecure or worthless. These are generally constituted by primary
maladaptive emotions of fear and shame.

Change, then, occurs by an important set of parallel processes.
The person accesses and symbolizes the expectancies associated with
the core emotion scheme. These are articulated as dysfunctional core
beliefs such as "I'm alone and unloved" or "I'm somehow contami-
nated—who would want me?" In addition, previously unacknowledged
or inaccessible primary adaptive emotions such as anger or disgust,
action tendencies, and the associated needs/goals for support or
protection are accessed and symbolized. These are used to develop a
sense of self-worth or security from which the client is enabled to
combat the articulated dysfunctional beliefs of the core maladaptive
scheme.

For example, the client mentioned above who kept looking for her
mother's love, when asked in a later session how she felt about her
mother's lack of contact, said, "I'm angry at her for continuing to be
so inconsiderate and selfish. I deserve a loving mother who appreciates
me. I refuse to put up with her behavior anymore, to be treated like a
doormat, taken for granted. I wouldn't put up with it from anyone
else." Or s client who had been sexually abused by a relative says, "I've
been ripped off, deprived of my childhood innocence. That's huge. I
hate him for doing this to me. And I hate my parents' refusal to talk
about it, making me suffer through this alone. I need them to be
outraged along with me, to want to support me, rather than shut me
down." Here the adaptive tendencies are strengthened by means of
shifting attention to internal resources and adaptive goals and by the
therapist's support of them. The newly accessed emotions and
needs/goals provide a new experience of self as well as challenges to
the dysfunctional beliefs. This results in a restructuring of the dysfunctional emotion schemes at the core of the disorder.

By arousing and "going into" previously avoided bad feelings such
as hopelessness, helplessness, feeling like a failure, or feeling alone and
abandoned, in the safety and comfort providing presence of another,
a number of things occur:

1. *The appraisals of self and situation* and *the associated action tendency*
involved in the initial emotional reaction are identified. Thus in
exploring a feeling of powerlessness a person might identify an appraisal—"Her cold stare spelled danger"; identify an emotional reac-

tion—"I felt so powerless and uncared for"; and an action tendency—"I just shrank inside and wanted to disappear" (Greenberg & Korman, 1993).

2. The *need/goal/concern* involved in the situation is also identified, as when the client says, "I needed her to acknowledge me—just to say, 'I see you exist.' " Once the appraisals, the needs to which they relate, and the action tendency have been identified, the picture or meaning of the client's experience becomes a lot clearer.

3. Having evoked the bad feeling, the *internal sequences* involved in generating the bad feeling become more accessible. Exploring these sequences finally accesses the *core maladaptive emotion scheme* and the associated expectancies that can be articulated as *beliefs*. Such a primary maladaptive emotion scheme is articulated as when the above client, after some exploration, says, "I feel like without her support I cease to exist, like I'm worthless unless I'm recognized."

4. Acknowledging this sense of insecurity and worthlessness makes this experience *amenable to new input*. Prior to its acknowledgement it is inaccessible, but once in awareness it is available for further processing. A new sense of self can now emerge.

Reorganization in the latter process occurs by a *shift* in attentional allocation or a change in perspective. The reorganization either occurs spontaneously and is supported by the therapist, for example, when a client says spontaneously, "I was not bad, I was a good little girl," or its emergence is facilitated by the therapist, both by guiding the client's attention to the emergence of some new need/goal and emotionally/motivationally based potential and by confirming the existence of internal resources as they emerge. The latter is done by attending to and validating these resources. Thus the therapist might hear in the client's momentary expression of anger the emergence of a sense of autonomy and a feeling of being able to separate and survive, and then might bring this into focal attention with a question such as "What are you feeling right now?" or an empathic response such as "I heard a flicker of strength in your voice." The above client who previously shrank away inside and felt worthless now contacts his strengths or internal resources and is able to feel, and say, "I can survive without her support. I know it won't be forever." Or a therapist's question, "What do you need?" in response to his feeling of sadness at being rejected, may help him access his alternate survival-oriented goals.

In the right facilitative environment, adaptive organismic concerns emerge in response to awareness of self-induced psychological distress that is internally generated. Guided by the person's motivation to survive, to cope, and to attach and seek contact/comfort, and supported by the therapist's empathic attunement to these, the client's adaptive emotions and needs are mobilized in response to felt suffering. Thus a person's need for support emerges in response to the experienced hostility and self-criticism of the internal critic. This occurs because criticism hurts. A clear example of this emerged in a student training session in which a trainee directed harsh criticisms at herself for being "lazy": "You'll never amount to anything. You're completely self-indulgent." She immediately burst into tears. In processing the experience, she said she felt the full impact of the criticisms and then felt her need for her own support and encouragement rather than the constant criticism.

Similarly, a need for rest often emerges in response to experiencing being overly driven by oneself, a need for self-preservation or strength often emerges in response to feeling battered by oneself, a need for comfort often arises in response to feeling abandoned, and a capacity to survive often emerges after one acknowledges that one feels shattered. What is needed is to pay attention to these healthy resources and thereby increase their role in the self-organizing process. For example, a client reliving the desperation of her abandonment by her husband some 20 years earlier wept deeply about never wanting to let herself be hurt again but followed this spontaneously with "But I am not a young dependent mother any more."

Alternate self-organizations constituted by adaptive organismic concerns and primary emotions therefore emerge in therapeutic environments that confirm them. These resources can then be used to combat the dysfunctional thoughts and beliefs involved in the bad feeling, or can be used to overcome the anxieties and fears of shattered attachments. The therapist's response to the above client's reworking of her supports captures the emergence of the client's strengths with "Yes, it so hurt to be so rejected, and you needed to feel safe, but it sounds like you're saying you're no longer defenseless. (C: Yeah.) Seems like you've learned a lot in the last 20 years about taking care of yourself."

Thus the process of change in working with bad feelings involves neither allowing and accepting them per se, nor insight, nor a new understanding, nor only being understood by another, nor simply a change in a belief. Rather, it involves a self-reorganization based on a newly accessed need/goal and emotional response that is strengthened by being supported and confirmed by another. From our study of transcripts of in-therapy change events, it is this increased accessibility to alternate aspects of self and self-reorganization around these new experiences that appears to be the key to change when one is dealing with bad feelings. We refer to this as *emotional restructuring* and see it as a crucial change process.

This type of emotional restructuring involves arousal of the core maladaptive emotional experience in the session and *in vivo* "hot" learning, in which a new emotional response is experienced in the session, one that counteracts the old maladaptive response. This results in change in core schemes and can often result in the resolution of complex difficulties.

Teaching Regulation and Coping Skills

A further goal is to teach skills of emotional regulation in order to help clients better deal with their bad feelings outside of therapy. This is done by facilitating experiential or "hot" learning about regulation in the context of aroused bad feeling, as opposed to "cool" learning of these skills in an instructional and conceptual manner. This teaching must therefore be in-therapy experiential teaching. This is best done when the relevant emotion state is currently aroused and is being experienced, or has just been experienced, in therapy. If a client feels overwhelmed and panicky in the session the therapist asks the client to breathe, to relax, and to continue to express his feelings. The client may then be encouraged to tell the therapist what he or she is afraid of, and to gradually approach the feared experience. Experiential teaching of regulation skills also involves helping people find ways, in the moment, of achieving appropriate distance from troubling emotions so as to be able to symbolize them and not be overwhelmed by them. Teaching emotion regulation involves teaching such skills as are described in the following subsections.

Attention Regulation Skills. Here people learn to focus on their present sensory awareness of internal and external reality rather than thoughts. People learn to focus in the session on the actual sensations and other constitutive elements of bad feelings such as action tendencies and muscular tension. This process provides training in coming into the present, in order to overcome dysfunctional ruminating and anticipating. Clients who are anxious or who are dissociating can be asked to look at the therapist or feel their feet on the floor in order to focus their attention on present sensory reality. Training in focusing on constituent elements of emotion such as breathing, tensing, and sensing also has the effect of destructuring or disrupting the automatic synthesis of bad feelings, thereby modifying those feelings for the present. This appears to work in a fashion similar to how attention to performance details of a complex skill destructures the skill, as when attending to the movement of the fingers in typing disrupts the higher level holistic performance. Thus, while feeling angry, if one attends to the heat in one's face, to one's jaw, to the clenching of the fist, and to one's breathing, the angry feeling begins to transform. Thus a variety of attentional control and meditational practices can be taught and practiced.

Breathing Regulation. This is one of the most crucial emotion regulation skills. When one is feeling bad feelings, breathing patterns are interfered with. Unaware, people hold their breath, they breath shallowly, or they hyperventilate. Paying attention to breathing focuses attention on current sensation, clears the mind of ruminations, and helps regulate breathing. This provides a very strong self-soothing effect. Thus as a client recalls terrifying beatings or another talks about the traumatic suicide of a parent, instructions to breath while talking about the experience can be very helpful.

Muscular Relaxation.   Breath regulation helps relaxation but explicit attention to tensing and relaxing muscles is also a helpful skill. Thus, clients with anxiety can benefit from engaging in relaxation exercises during the session, particularly when they are tense or are talking about an anxiety-provoking situation.

Self-Nurturing and Other Emotion Regulation Coping Skills. Self-soothing skills associated with breathing are taught. This involves developing compassion and empathy for the self that is in distress. Self-empathy and -compassion are explicitly taught as well as shaped and encouraged. "Here and now" skills, such as the above, are taught in conjunction with encouragement to engage in behaviors such as taking a walk or a bath, reading, listening to music, or in some way taking care of oneself to help one deal with bad feelings. These can be important educative aspects of an emotionally focused treatment for helping people cope with bad feelings outside of therapy. It is ideal to engage in some small form of practice of this in the session before giving extrasessional homework. For example, a client can practice paying attention to what he or she needs in the moment and imagining getting it, or giving it to oneself, or planning how to do it after the session.

In an example of self-nurturing homework a client, after intense exploration of painful material, says, "I just want to shut down, not think anymore. I feel tired and drained." The therapist reflects this need for rest and asks if there will be an opportunity to do this, to go home and take a warm bath or do something soothing. In working with trauma clients who are often avoidant of experience, it is also good to talk about appropriate avoidance and shutting down, about when to *choose* to do this in order to take care of oneself.

The Process of Working with Painful Experience

Allowing pain and acceptance of it are similar to working with bad feelings, in that the feelings need to be approached rather than avoided. Pain differs, however, in that it is the "facing" or "feeling through" of the feelings, such as loss or grief, that results in its resolution by means of further emotional processing. Facing pain does not involve as much exploration and unpacking of the complex meanings nor the accessing of dysfunctional core emotion schemes as does therapeutic work with bad feelings. Nor does facing pain necessarily involve the same type of reorganization. Rather, facing painful feelings requires overcoming the fear that the self may be shattered so that the pain is allowed and the traumatic material is assimilated. Emotional processing in the allowing of pain, then, is a type of exposure treatment—exposure to the pain in order to change elements of the pain-producing structure (Foa & Kozak, 1986; Greenberg & Safran, 1984a, 1984b, 1987). This can be followed by meaning reconstruction in which dysfunctional beliefs associated with the pain are changed from "It's humiliating to be needy" to "I really need contact and can learn to get these needs met."

Solutions to the problems of pain do not lie in understanding the sources of the pain or the losses suffered, which often are only too evident. Rather, change comes by allowing and accepting the pain, which has been avoided in an attempt to protect the self, and by experiencing and expressing the feelings in order to live them through to completion. Events that are experienced as traumatic often result in the emotions generated by the event being denied so that the person is left feeling numb. The internal operations of interrupting highly aroused emotion at the time of trauma are designed to control potentially overwhelming affects that, although generally useful in enabling rapid adaptive action, are at that time no longer perceived to be adaptive. It is the persistence of the interruptive controls after the traumatic event has ceased and the continued avoidance that then become problematic.

For example, a client who had been traumatized as a child by repeatedly watching his mother being brutalized recalled an incident in which he wanted to kill his father and actually unsuccessfully looked for his father's gun. As a boy, he was powerless to do anything about the situation and his only recourse was to numb himself. As an adult, he felt distant from his own feelings, alienated from others, and suffered chronic depression. He had been unable to grieve over his mother's death and was distant from his own children. In therapy collaborative goals were to help him learn how to feel again. This involved feeling the hurt and anger he felt as a little boy, but at the same time accessing his adult resources.

The transformation that occurs in undoing overcontrol and allowing painful feelings has been one of the most undocumented mysteries of psychological healing and has led to the great controversy over the concept of catharsis. Our investigation suggests that the cathartic process of resolving pain is a complex one involving a variety of processes that can result in both relief and enduring change. Although allowing and accepting painful feelings relies on some organismic muscular release and neurochemical recuperative process (experienced as the ability to "go on," having suffered the pain), it is also important to recognize that it is not just the relief and release that leads to change. This experience also involves a cognitive change. It involves first a change in the ability to put previously inarticulate episodic memories into language. This facilitates gaining access to and control over them. In addition, it involves a change in the belief that the pain will destroy the self, as well as a change in certain expectancies or assumptions about oneself and the world, formed at the time of trauma. Feeling painful feelings, when therapeutic, thus involves both emotional release and relief, on the one hand, and cognitive change, on the other. The combination of all these changes results in a strengthened sense of self.

A Model for Resolving Painful Emotion

Based on our initial analysis of a number of episodes of therapeutic resolution of painful experience (Greenberg & Safran, 1987), we have progressively refined a model that depicts the in-therapy performance components of pain-resolution episodes. This is shown in Figure 5.3. As this model of the therapeutic resolution of painful experience shows, acknowledging the painful feelings is an early step in the process of change. At this stage, the previously avoided painful feelings must be *approached*, then *allowed*, and then *accepted* as part of oneself. In allowing the feeling of devastation, helplessness, or powerlessness, the original trauma has to be experienced and faced in order to know experientially that one can survive the pain. The acceptance of the pain offers a form of containment that helps to create a safe distance from the feeling and allows the need or affective goal associated with the feeling to be recognized and mobilized. This empowers the organism to combat any dysfunctional appraisals that are preventing and/or causing the pain. Allowing of the pain results in an organismic sense of relief and enables the person to emerge in a new self-affirming manner. The act of confronting traumatic memories has been found to reduce the physiological and cognitive work involved in inhibiting trauma-related thoughts and feelings (Pennebaker, 1989).

The critical sequence shown in Figure 5.3—allowing and accepting the pain, and of increasing the sense of agency by willingly experiencing the pain rather than feeling like a victim of it—results in a reowning and reassimilation of the painful experience. This change in internal relations helps the person mobilize previously unmet needs. It also helps to challenge the cognitions and beliefs that are involved in the pain and its interruption, and to transform them. It is once again the mobilization of previously inaccessible resources of the essential self, such as the inherent desire for mastery, the exploratory curiosity, or the desire for attachment (all of which can be viewed as the will to live), that are transformative. This process of facing pain, accessing needs, and combating dysfunctional beliefs results both in a sense of relief and the adoption of a more self-nurturing and self-affirming stance.

From a phenomenological perspective, when people deal with core dreaded painful aspects of self, they learn that they can survive what they previously believed was unendurable. They metaphorically face their own existential death and are reborn. It is of interest to note that the powerless, helpless feeling in pain is not the same as the secondary helplessness of depression or anxiety. The latter has to be overcome, but the former is a primary state to be acknowledged, faced, and coped with, rather than avoided.

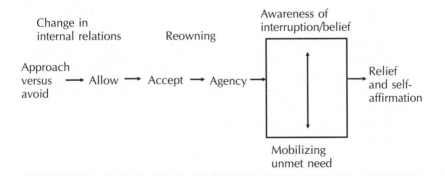

FIGURE 5.3. Allowing of painful experience.

Facing pain involves a type of exposure treatment, with three critical differences to the original behavioral approach. First, facing painful feelings is exposure to previously avoided *internal* experience rather than to an avoided external stimulus. Second, there is a change in *meaning* rather than a change in conditioning. Third, *novelty* is introduced by accessing new internal affective information and resources rather than by engaging in a new behavior. For example, a client who had lost her infant faced her dreaded sense of internal rupture and brokenness in therapy, as well as her shame at having left the hospital before her baby's death. She forgave herself for not being able to endure the pain and saw her whole life since then as a struggle to protect herself against the pain. In finally facing her pain, she decided to face life, to face living again, rather than to protect herself behind a wall of fear.

With acceptance of previously avoided feeling and with survival, people no longer rigidly attend to threat cues signaling the emergence of the dreaded feeling so they can avoid or escape them. They are more flexible and open to new information and the feelings have less power over them. The conditions and opportunity for novelty, for seeing new possibilities, and creating new meaning now exist.

EFT directs clients' attention to their internal experience. This helps them to access new internal resources, previously inaccessible, and to look for novel ways of coping. It is the *shift* to accessing organismic needs, as well as the motivation of the essential self to survive and grow, that provides a basis for novel coping. Knowing what one wants and needs empowers the individual to become an agent on her or his own behalf in obtaining needed support and nurturance. Nurturing and support can be obtained both internally, in the form of self soothing and self-valuing, and interactionally. Clients can receive validation and support from the therapist and can act in the world to obtain support by self-assertively asking others for it or defining their boundaries.

This process of allowing and accepting pain therefore requires that it be evoked in the session and lived through, not talked about. By experiencing the pain in its actuality, you are in essence in a novel situation in which you learn that the pain is endurable and will not destroy you. In addition, you are then opened to new possibilities and can attend to new information. This new experience restructures the pain-producing emotional schemes.

Two sources of new experience in the here and now of the therapy session are essential in dealing with the pain. First, the safe, valuing presence of the therapist provides comfort and validation, and this function is partially internalized (Greenberg et al., 1993). Second, a new perspective is created. The client develops a new place to stand from which to view the painful experience and how it was created. With the help of these two aids, interpersonal support and an internal shift in perspective, one is able to establish a working distance from what was previously overwhelming and access a more self-nurturing and self-affirming set of functions. A description of the development of this nurturing stance was provided by a client who, for research purposes, watched a videotape of herself struggling with deeply painful material and described her experience at the time. Watching herself on tape, the client said she could see how hard this woman was struggling and that her heart went out to her. She said that for the first time in her life, she felt great empathy for herself and her own pain.

This move to more positive coping is in part governed by the organism's tendency to "go on" and to seek more positive, comfortable, adaptive states rather than stay in pain. The paradox is that avoidance of the aversiveness of pain perpetuates it and interferes with the ability to move away from it. One needs to embrace the pain, to face the hopeless, helpless feeling being staved off, and to truly move on from it by restructuring it. This is what is meant by the colloquial terms "going into" and "going through" pain, in which the emergence of newness is captured by the mythic image of the phoenix rising from the ashes. In this image, organization emerges out of disorganization and destruction. In working with pain, therapists therefore need to promote the above steps of resolving it by helping clients attend to, approach, and symbolize their painful experience. Therapists need to encourage acceptance of that experience, and they need to facilitate agency or reowning of it. EFT does not promote retraumatization but creates a safe environment in which clients allow themselves to experience their pain in order to heal.

THE CENTRALITY OF ALLOWING IN EMOTION WORK

Although emotion operates in different ways at different times in the therapeutic change process (Greenberg & Safran, 1987; Greenberg et al., 1993), allowing previously disallowed emotion is one key aspect that operates throughout. Again, allowing emotional experience in therapy appears to facilitate change by changing internal relations, reowning, and increasing a sense of agency.

The change in internal relations involves a move from avoidance and negative evaluation of internal experience to an *accepting* stance.

Painful, bad, and hopeless feelings are not "things as such," but products of internal relations. Thus, vulnerability that is unacceptable becomes panic, anger that is unacceptable becomes alienation or despair, and unacceptable loss becomes struggle. When acknowledged, vulnerability or anger become information and internal resources. The very acts of approaching, attending to, and accepting or positively evaluating feelings leads to their transformation. Emotionally reengaging previously disowned emotional experience promotes assimilation. In evoking and allowing the experience, emotion memory is fully activated, arraying in consciousness more of the experience where it can be symbolized in awareness and made more comprehensible (Greenberg & Pascual-Leone, 1995).

Facing hopelessness is often a key phase in the allowing and acceptance process. Although certain forms of hopelessness such as depressive feelings of desperate powerlessness are often secondary feelings that need to be bypassed or explored, accepting other forms of hopelessness is a crucial first step in change. Giving up a useless struggle against feeling hopeless and allowing yourself to experience and face your avoided hopelessness is essential to change. Facing this hopelessness, rather than avoiding it, involves a paradoxical change process. Generally it appears that hopelessness is undesirable, that therapy is geared toward engendering hope, and that it is good to feel hopeful. If, however, we are able to give up struggling against the inevitable and accept the feeling of hopelessness, this will lead us to letting go of unworkable strategies or unattainable goals. Hopelessness in these situations does not mean depression or despair. Rather, it is acceptance of what cannot be avoided, enabling one to begin to take responsibility for new efforts and new goals. Hopelessness thus involves giving up futile efforts and reorganizing. Facing hopelessness is not believing that "I am hopeless" but that a particular effort is not working and that my efforts to overcome are of no avail. Contacting and accepting the experience of the futility of the struggle is often a critical step in an emotional change process. This involves facing what has been fearfully avoided, letting go of unworkable solutions, and setting the stage for creative reorganization.

Reowning is the second important process. It involves identifying with feelings and associated thoughts, memories, needs, and action tendencies that have been disowned. Disowned experience, although not integrated into the dominant self-organization, still do exert influence on behavior. People tend to deal with the unacceptable by depersonalizing their feelings and not experiencing them as their own, thus weakening their self-organization. Thus therapy can be understood not as a process of bringing previously unconscious material into consciousness but as one of *reclaiming disowned experience*. One can also distinguish between the conceptual processing of information in an intellectual way and the experiential linking of that information to the self (Greenberg et al., 1993). It is the latter that is important in reowning and therapeutic change.

Acknowledging pain or dreaded feelings is then the first step in a problem-solving process in which identifying such feelings is akin to problem definition. The person identifies in an experientially valid fashion that the problem is that "I feel rotten, powerless, or unlovable" or that "My heart is broken—I don't wish to carry on." You cannot leave a place until you have arrived at that place, and so it is with dreaded feelings. It is the experiencing of the distressing feeling that makes it unequivocally clear what the problem is and thus is a key ingredient in motivating new ways of coping with that feeling. Rather than the old style of alternately avoiding or feeling overwhelmed and out of control and sinking into despair, numbness, depression, and anxiety, the client, in the safe and supportive therapeutic situation, is able to process more information. She or he is able to bring previously unused resources to bear on coping with the distress-producing condition.

For example, a client who, for the first time, accessed in therapy a traumatic experience associated with sexual abuse felt the intense pain of shame, plus the deep sadness at her loss of innocence. Supported by the therapist she felt empathy for herself as a little girl, and quickly switched to intense anger at the perpetrator for ripping her off. The therapist empathically responded to her vulnerability and validated her experience of being violated. At the end of the session, the client remarked that despite the pain, she felt hopeful that "things will change," adding "I at least feel like these feelings are my own and I have a right to feel them."

This client's comments also illustrate the increased sense of *agency* that emerges from the above two processes. With reowning comes an increased sense of self in relation to a domain of experience. Gestalt therapists (Perls, 1973; Yontef & Simkins, 1989) use deliberate awareness experiments to promote experiences of agency in which the person experiences that *"It is I who is thinking, feeling, needing, wanting, or doing this."* Hope develops, from the sense that "It is *I* who is feeling this, it is me who is an agent in this feeling" and then "It is me who can do something about this." A sense of agency is created by recognizing oneself as a creator or author of one's experience. While a sense of agency may not yet provide a concrete plan of action, there is a feeling of confidence that action is possible and that change can occur.

GENERAL PROCESSES

A Dialectical Process

Part of the complexity in describing how change occurs through expression and exploration of emotion is that change often involves a dialectical process of small step-by-step increments in the integration of conceptual and experiential processing. Change needs to be viewed as part of the ongoing functioning of a dynamic system that operates by the dialectical synthesis of components in an ongoing self-organizing process. Highlighting of any element by attentional allocation or symbolization, or the introduction of new information, acts as a perturbation to the system, which reorganizes around the new element. Two principles of emotional change stated by Greenberg and Safran (1987) sought to describe this process. One, the principle that in emotional change one thing follows another incrementally, captured the dynamic ongoing process of reorganization. The second, the polarity principle, captured that a dialectical synthesis of elements drives this process.

Small Steps

In addition, if dreaded bad feelings rush in too quickly and overwhelm, people will tighten against these feelings, fearing dissolution. Their inability to control their feelings will leave them diminished in their sense of agency and ability to control themselves. If, however, the experience of the feelings are regulated such that the person's sense of control is not undermined, or if sufficient support is present to accept some letting go of control and regaining it, then change occurs. For example, in working with abuse survivors and using an empty-chair dialogue to evoke trauma memories and experience, we have found it helpful to have the client first confront a nonthreatening other, such as her or his nonprotective mother. She or he tells the story of the abuse in this context before directly confronting the perpetrator (Paivio, Lake, Nieuwenhuis, & Baskerville, 1996).

Thus emotional reprocessing by graded exposure to optimal levels of arousal is most helpful in promoting change. In this process a safe supportive environment is essential in providing some form of containment. Containment here does not mean prevention or dampening of experience but rather providing an environment that helps to hold the feelings, allowing them to be, but not to escalate or run away. People also need to feel they can let themselves experience their feelings at a pace and in a manner that is not too overwhelming and when they have sufficient internal strength and support to assimilate them. In this case acknowledgment of the bad feeling is accompanied by a type of relief rather than panic.

Symbolizing Feelings

The ability to reprocess emotion by attaching words to feelings introduces new elements of meaning and also gives a person a sense of control. Symbolization provides a handle on the feeling and thereby modifies it. Thus a client who symbolizes her feeling as "I feel so left out" when talking about social conversations is able to say, "I'm trying so hard to keep up, but actually I'm often not interested. That's why I've nothing to say." Another client symbolizes her experiences as "I feel like there's a ghost in the room and I can never fill her shoes" when talking about taking over from a previous supervisor. She then acknowledges, "I can't do what she did. I'm different and will use my own strengths." Symbolization promoted the generation of new meaning.

In addition, symbolization of experience creates a stronger sense of self because, by being able to denote feeling, an act of separation from it occurs. By linguistically symbolizing emotion, one has in effect simultaneously created a new place to stand, a new perspective from which to see the feeling as well as provide a label for the feeling itself, thereby knowing what one feels. It is now "I" who feels "this," and this is separate from me. This provides an organized experience of a coherent self as an "agent" experiencing a nameable feeling, rather than being a passive victim of the feeling. This establishment of a self in relation to the feeling is a relationship that provides the self with a sense both of coherence and agency. Thus symbolizing that "I feel like a failure," although painful, also produces solidity and promotes coping.

Change from, say, self-condemnation to self-support involves first experiencing the bad feeling, then symbolizing it to yourself, and then reflexively reviewing your view (Watson & Greenberg, 1995; Greenberg & Pascual-Leone, 1997). These processes of arousing, symbolizing, and reflecting help access self support and counteract the bad feeling until system reorganization occurs (Greenberg et al., 1993; Greenberg & Pascual-Leone, 1995; Watson & Greenberg, 1995). Thus a client talking in a session about not getting a promotion began to feel hopeless about ever furthering his career. After expressing self-criticisms he focused internally and said, "I feel like there's a good chance I won't ever reach the top." Although revealing disappointment, this acknowledgment brought him a sense of relief and calm, and he began to talk about early retirement and doing some of the things he had always wanted to do. Thus he began reordering his priorities.

In addition, people who have suffered trauma and endured deeply painful experiences can begin a reconstructive process of assimilating the trauma by putting it into language. The capacity to symbolize emotionally traumatic experience permits the articulation, literally the making sense of, what previously were ineffable and inarticulate qualities of the experience. By evoking memories that carry traumatic emotional content and symbolizing this in a safe environment, people gain control over their experience and become authors rather than victims of that experience.

The Self as an Agent in the Construction of Bad Feelings

An additional way of empowering the self in the process of dealing with previously avoided bad feeling is to highlight the role of the self in the creation of the bad feeling while accessing that feeling. Thus, people can feel rotten and worthless or dependent and despairing and also experience in awareness how they create the feeling by an internal process of criticizing and condemning the self, or by terrifying themselves and undermining their sense of security. They then experience that they are "making" themselves feel rotten and unlovable.

For example, exploring a client's conflict between fearing and desiring an intimate relationship, the therapist tentatively suggests, "It sounds like you're saying they always let you down but that you somehow bring it on, (C: Yeah.) that there's something fundamentally wrong with you. . . . What, (C: Yeah.) I wonder, are you implicitly saying to yourself, is wrong with you, and why it is you can't have a relationship?" It is crucial to note that this type of intervention is not one of blaming the person for making themselves feel bad but rather helping them to see how their bad feeling is constructed. Therapist manner and style are therefore crucial in this intervention, with nonjudgmentalness and validation of the client's experience being crucial. Acknowledgement that the negative messages clients give themselves are often internalized from their families of origin is helpful in alleviating further self-blame. Moreover, they learn that automatic processes that are learned can be unlearned, and this enhances agency. Once people are able to see themselves as agents in producing bad feeling, the experience of feeling rotten and unlovable has already changed. Once again, a different perspective has been created.

CONCLUSION

Change through feeling involves a complex set of emotional and cognitive processes and requires a variety of different types of interventions to change these. This is not a process of cathartic dumping of emotions. The term "differentiating feelings" is used to describe the complex process of emotional exploration. This is a condensed term for all the processes mentioned above, which result in the symbolization of differentiated facets of experience, integration of these different facets into new meaning, and reflexive operations to create new meaning.

CHAPTER SIX

The Phases of Emotionally Focused Intervention

IN THIS CHAPTER we will outline the phases of intervention. This approach has not been devised for, or applied to, psychotic or psychopathic populations, people with high suicidal risk, or other highly functionally impaired populations whose predominant psychotherapeutic needs may be for coping skills or other forms of support or intervention. It has been designed and proved effective with clients who are depressed and anxious and suffer from interpersonal problems, childhood maltreatment, and problems in living (Greenberg & Watson, in press; Paivio & Greenberg, 1995). We will begin by briefly overviewing the steps of this approach to intervention and identifying the intervention principles that guide therapist's intentions and actions. This is followed by a detailed discussion of the steps in emotionally focused therapy (EFT).

The first step in this treatment involves forming a supportive relationship by acknowledging, understanding, and validating the client's emotional struggles. When the client feels understood, he or she will form an emotional bond, a critical element in the development of an alliance. Acknowledgment of feeling also establishes an early focus on the client's internal experience and on the emotional impact of environmental and interpersonal events.

As the therapy proceeds the therapist continually focuses on the difficult or painful feelings and uses empathic reflections to underscore the emotional impact of experience. A consistent and gentle pressure is thus applied, in a highly supportive context, to help the person get closer and closer to that "bad feeling experience in there," to feeling "heavy," "hurt," "desperate" or "in conflict." Thus right from the start there is an implicit training in focusing on internal experience and on facing, rather than avoiding, painful experience (Gendlin, 1981, 1996; Klein, Mathieu, Kiesler, & Gendlin, 1969).

After establishing an initial empathic bond, the therapist collaborates with the client to identify and develop a focus on the specific determinants of the client's painful and uncomfortable experience. Both client and therapist begin to understand that the client has some particular issue that affects the client's ability to regulate his or her own affect. Problems such as being unaware of feelings, as evaluating feelings negatively, as being in conflict, as having unresolved bad feelings, as resentment toward significant others, or as being unable to regulate closeness in relationships are seen as the source of distress. It may take a few sessions to develop and establish a focus, or core issues may be obvious right from the start.

Once the therapist and client have established an alliance and a focus, the therapist then concentrates on the affective component of the client's problematic experience. Therapy follows a sequence of evoking the bad feelings, exploring these feelings and their determinants, accessing primary emotions or core maladaptive emotion schemes, and then using newly accessed resources to facilitate reorganization of core schemes. The sequence ends with affirming and validating the emerging sense of self and consolidating change in a new identity narrative.

After the generating conditions or core issues are established, the aim is to evoke the negative experience or bad feeling (e.g., hopelessness or helplessness) so that it is lived in the session and, once evoked, to differentiate and explore the determinants of the secondary bad feeling or face the painful experience. In exploring the determinants of bad feeling, the aim is to tease out the different components of the experience until one accesses core maladaptive emotion schemes generating the bad feelings, such as feeling worthless or insecure, and/or alternate primary adaptive emotions, such as sadness at loss, anger at violation, or adaptive fear, and the needs or affective goals associated with these. Therapist responses at this point must highlight the emergence of such adaptive needs as needs for closeness, firmer boundaries, safety, or connectedness to act as the basis for adaptive alternatives to the core maladaptive schemes.

Accessing primary emotional experience that has been interrupted or not attended to helps identify new affective goals and produces a marked shift in organization. It produces a shift from hopelessness to a will to live, from helplessness to strength, from fear to assertive anger. These newly accessed primary, biologically adaptive feelings and the associated needs/goals/concerns are then used to challenge maladaptive cognitions, restructure maladaptive schemes, and act as the basis of new self-organizations. Finally, the therapist helps to validate self-affirmations and to help the client consolidate new meanings in a new narrative construction. The eight-step sequence that describes this process is spelled out more fully below.

The process of treatment is not a linear one in which client and therapist move one step at a time through the sequence. Rather, clients work at their own pace circling through the steps. The steps occur in stages only in the sense that each step or process depends on the previous one being attained to some degree. The therapist's style is not instructional nor interpretive; rather, it is facilitative of exploration and supports the emergence of new information through new experience. The therapist and client always collaborate in establishing momentary foci and in formulating and testing experientially grounded hypotheses and in coming to an agreement about goals and specific tasks.

Throughout, the therapist's intentions, guiding his or her actions, are those at the basis of an emotionally focused approach (Greenberg & Safran, 1987; Greenberg & Johnson, 1988). As shown in Table 6.1, these include the nine specific intentions of attending, refocusing, present-centeredness, expression analysis, promoting ownership, intensifying, memory evocation, symbolization, and establishment of intents, as well as the two more global intentions of balancing leading and following, and being emotionally present in a genuinely facilitative manner and making contact. The latter involves disclosing and using aspects of self- experience that emerge in the relationship in order to validate the client and promote exploration. These will be exemplified throughout subsequent chapters. The phases of treatment and the major steps in each phase are detailed below.

The framework for the process of EFT is presented in Table 6.2. The eight-step sequence is broken into three phases: the bonding phase, the evocation and exploration phase, and the emotion-restructuring phase. The first phase involves (1) attending to, empathizing with, and validating the client's feelings and current sense of self and (2) establishing a collaborative focus on generating conditions. The second phase involves (3) evoking and arousing problematic feelings and (4) exploring and unpacking cognitive–affective sequences generating experience. The third, emotion- restructuring phase involves the following steps: (5) accessing core maladaptive emotion schemes and/or primary adaptive emotions; (6) restructuring of core maladaptive schemes by facilitating challenge of maladaptive beliefs by primary emotion and newly emerged needs/goals; (7) validating new feelings and supporting an emerging sense of self; and (8) creating new meaning.

TABLE 6.1. Therapist Intentions and Actions

Specific intentions	Actions
1. Direct attention.	Respond empathically. Direct attention.
2. Refocus attention.	Redirect attention to internal experiential track.
3. Focus on present.	Bring clients' attention to present experience.
4. Analyze expression.	Comment in a supportive manner on, and create awareness of nonverbal expression. Focus on how things are said.
5. Promote ownership and agency.	Promote use of "I" language speaking as disowned parts. Reown experience.
6. Intensify.	Use vivid imagery and expressive enactments. Suggest exaggerations and repetition of expressions and actions.
7. Evoke memories.	Promote reentry and reliving of concrete events of the past from the client's point of view. Focus on emotional content of memories, personal perceptions, and meanings.
8. Symbolize.	Put feelings into words mainly by empathic responses. Conjecture on what might be felt. Promote reflection and creation of new meaning.
9. Establish intents.	Focus on wants, needs, and goals by asking what do you need. Promote planning and action in the world.

Global intentions	Actions
1. Balance leading and following.	Many varied actions.
2. Be present and make contact.	Many varied actions.

PHASE I: BONDING

Attend, Empathize, and Validate

In the initial stages of therapy the goals are to make contact with the client and to establish a warm, empathic, and collaborative bond. This helps the client to feel understood, relax, and focus internally. The therapist attends to the client's experience and becomes empathically attuned to the client's feelings. The client is implicitly trained to attend

TABLE 6.2. The Framework

Phase I: Bonding

1. Attend to, empathize, and validate feelings. Convey understanding of client's bad feelings or painful experience and validate how painful and difficult the struggle is.

2. Establish and develop a collaborative focus. Identify the underlying cognitive–affective processes or generating conditions. Identify as foci of therapeutic work such generating conditions as self-criticism or dependence and interpersonal loss.

Phase II: Evoking and exploring

3. Evocation and arousal. The bad feeling or painful experience is brought alive in the session or regulated.

4. Explore/unpack cognitive affective sequences in the painful experience or that generate the bad feelings.

Phase III: Emotion restructuring

5. Access the core maladaptive emotion scheme and/or primary emotional experience.

6. Restructure. Facilitate restructuring of core schemes by challenging maladaptive beliefs with newly accessed primary adaptive needs/goals and resources. Support emergence of primary needs/goals and emotional resources.

7. Support and validate emergence of a more self-affirming stance. Support mobilization of resources, self-soothing capacities, improved affect regulation, and self-empathy.

8. Creation of new meaning. Promote reflection. Construct a new narrative and new metaphors to capture new meanings.

to internal experience by the therapist's empathic responses, which consistently focuses on the client's internal experience. The therapist conveys understanding, acknowledges the client's pain, validates his or her struggles, and focuses on the emotional impact of events in the client's life.

A good example of the importance of this attending process occurred in supervision with a novice therapist. A client who was diabetic came to her initial therapy sessions with long, detailed stories of her medication and her trips to the doctor. Her novice therapist tried to follow the content and details and sequence and became impatient because the client was "storytelling" and not on topic about core material. The therapist failed to hear in the client's voice her impatience at having to exercise such control in her life. The therapist also missed the message when the client said, almost in passing, "Sometimes, I can't bear to take another pill." A more attuned therapist might respond, "You're fed up to the eyeballs with this constant self-monitoring and control." Such a response would help the client feel understood and focus on important internal experience and unmet needs. Thus the therapist establishes the focus on emotional experience and simultaneously validates and supports the client's feelings with statements such as "I hear how heavy this is," "It's so difficult to fail," "What a struggle this is," "I see the tears behind the laugh," "It still really stings," "It's hard to feel so over-whelmed," or "You're just at your wit's end." Here validation confirms the clients emotional reality.

When clients talk about their week or about past events, the therapist attends to their present emotional experience and responds empathically. Statements that validate and underscore affective experience also help to evoke emotional reactions in the session. When therapists reflect how hard it must be, tears will often well up in clients' eyes and they will begin to open up about their experience, or they will visibly suppress their experience. In either case, these are important markers of current cognitive–affective processes that the therapist will be attuned to and will validate by saying, "It hurts to think about those things" or "It's really hard to feel those things."

From the very first session, therapist responses focus on and reiterate the importance of client emotional experience. Problems are defined in feeling terms. The bodily felt sense is attended to, with the goal of accessing the emotion scheme that generates personal emotional meaning. Eventually such a focus helps clients attend to, acknowledge (overcome avoidance), and fully experience their own painful feelings and emotional meanings in the safety of the therapeutic environment. Once these feelings are out in the open, alternate needs/goals/concerns are accessed, internal resources can be brought to bear, experience can be differentiated, clarified, and understood, and dysfunctional processes can be collaboratively modified.

Some clients are extremely externally focused, and helping them contact their feelings can be challenging. A persistent gentle pressure to focus on current internal experience is required by means, first, of empathic responding and questions and, later, by process directives that focus attention on internal experience. Only later can process directives can be used to stimulate emotion in the session. A balance needs to be struck between allowing clients to tell their story and express their reactions, on the one hand, and explicitly directing their attention internally, on the other.

Develop a Focus on Generating Conditions

A defining feature of emotionally focused intervention is that it is process diagnostic (Greenberg et al., 1993). There is a continual focus on the client's current cognitive–affective problem and state and the identification of markers of current emotional concerns. This guides intervention. It is the client's presently felt experience that indicates what the difficulty is and whether problem determinants are currently accessible and amenable to intervention. The early establishment of a focus and of generating conditions acts only as a broad framework to initially focus exploration. The focus is always subject to change and development, and process diagnosis of in-session problems states always acts as a major means of focusing each session.

Identifying and articulating the problematic cognitive–affective processes underlying and generating the client's surface bad feelings is a collaborative effort between the therapist and client. This helps alliance development in that it implicitly suggests that the goal of the treatment, or this phase of it, is to resolve this issue. An explicit agreement is often established that treatment goals involve addressing these conditions.

It is at this stage that a statement of and an agreement on the goals of treatment emerge. These goals are based on the therapist and client developing understanding of the generating conditions of the client's problems. Thus a goal for a depressed client might be to acknowledge and stand up to his overly hostile self-critic, which produces feelings of inadequacy. For another client with low self-esteem the goal might be to be more aware of, and more clearly able to express, her feelings and needs. For another dependent client the goal might be to assertively express and resolve her resentment at feeling dominated by her husband. For an anxious client a goal might be to develop a means of self-soothing and self-support; for another, to calm her anxiety, or to restructure a deep fear of abandonment and insecurity based on traumas or losses in the past. This clarification of specific and personal problem generators is an important aspect of establishing a good collaborative alliance, as is a formulation of relevant goals.

For example, a client entered therapy complaining that she was too timid and unclear about what she was feeling. The therapist responded, "It seems that one of the things you'd like to accomplish in therapy is to feel a stronger sense of yourself, so you can stand up for yourself." When the client agreed, the therapist discussed how they might accomplish this in therapy. The therapist suggested they might use active tasks in the session to help her explore her internal experience and that this would help her to more clearly understand what she was feeling, thinking, and needing. The encapsulation of the problem also makes the client feel deeply understood, and this enhances the bond. Note that it is implicit or explicit *agreement* on goals that is important in the establishment of the alliance, not the setting of goals per se. Thus goals can be implicit as long as there is a sense of shared goals and collaboration ensues. This step of developing a focus has three aspects: identifying a specific type of generating condition, developing awareness of agency in the creation of the generating condition, and using the generating condition to help provide a treatment rationale.

Identify the Type of Generating Conditions

Research on a large sample of emotionally focused interventions revealed that we focus on three basic types of generating conditions: (1) difficulties in symbolizing internal experience; (2) problematic relations between aspects of self; or (3) problematic relations between self and other (Goldman, 1995). Although determinants are unique for each person, many can be broadly grouped into these nonmutually exclusive clusters. Working with symbolization involves helping clients attend to, symbolize, and reflect on bodily felt experience to generate new meaning. Working on problematic self–self relations involves resolving issues of self-definition and self-esteem, such as being overly self-critical or perfectionistic. Working on problematic interpersonal relations often involves issues related to attachment and interdependence problems, such as feeling too dependent or too vulnerable to rejection. The latter two categories cohere with current views by a number of theorists on the importance of both intrapsychic and interpersonal problems in dysfunction (Blatt & Mouradas, 1992). Resolving issues of self-definition and attachment and balancing needs for separateness and connectedness appear to be core human tasks.

Symbolizing Internal Experience. The first task is helping the client focus on internal experience by means of exploration, attentional focusing, and evocative responding. Through this process clients become aware of and symbolize their previously unacknowledged feelings and emotions. Here the client task is one of vividly reentering the lived situation in an attempt to reexperience, more fully and with more attentional allocation, the emotional responses and the associated appraisals, needs, and action tendencies.

In the process of identifying generating conditions, the therapist's actions are intended predominantly to refocus the client on internal experience. It is important here for the therapist to distinguish between clients' *primary affective responses* to situations and their *secondary reactions* to their more primary responses and to continually focus toward primary experience and its symbolization. For example, a client's secondary reaction to a primary feeling of fear of abandonment might be anger at him- or herself for feeling afraid or angry at another for distancing. Therapists need to consistently focus on symbolizing the more primary response. Thus, although the therapist would acknowledge a client's secondary reactive anger at the self or the other, the major thrust of the therapist's response will focus on symbolizing the client's primary fear of abandonment.

Because emotions can be experienced as unlabeled and unarticulated feeling states, therapists and clients should not rely solely on talking as a means of identifying and dealing with emotion in therapy. They should also use attentional allocation, expressive behavior, and body sensation occurring in the session to help identify and ultimately symbolize emotions. EFT does not rely heavily on direct questions such as "What are you feeling." We have found that these questions can heighten defensiveness in clients who are already anxious, and many clients are not clear on what they are feeling. It is preferable therefore to tentatively and empathically respond to feelings, or to conjecture about what clients may be feeling. This helps clients feel understood and educates them in emotion awareness and the process of exploration. If a conjecture is offered tentatively, it enables clients to say, "No, not really angry, just kind of frustrated. . . ."

Identifying Intrapersonal Determinants. The following are some of the key self–self relations focused on in the EFT approach:

1. *Chronic overcontrol and lack of awareness of feeling.* As discussed in Chapter 4 on the sources of emotional disorder, some clients habitually constrict their emotional experience and expression and are cut off from their feelings or from specific classes of feelings. In the therapy session one can observe extreme avoidance strategies or defenses such as numbing or disassociation, or more moderate avoidant processes such as lack of experiential awareness and distracting. Again active suppression of emotional experience often occurs in clients who view some aspect of the experience as threatening or unacceptable. For example, a client who learned that her anger toward her parents jeopardized the needed relationship with them suppressed her anger. Another client, who had been raped as an adolescent, learned to use chronic anger and sexual "distractions" to distance himself from painful hurt and shame. The task here is one of increasing clients' awareness of how they interrupt and avoid their feelings in the session and helping them overcome these blocks.

2. *Conflict between aspects of the self.* This is manifested either in conflict between two aspects of self, such as "I want to tell him what I think but I'm afraid to," or in the form of self-criticism, self-doubt, negative self-evaluation, or internal threats to self-esteem (Greenberg,

1984; Greenberg et al., 1993). The latter experiences involve some form of negative statements inflicted on the self. Statements are inflicted either with hostility and the belief that whipping the self into shape will be helpful or to protect the self by being overly vigilant and monitoring and cautioning the self. Many people in therapy feel that they are fundamentally unacceptable or that their deeds, thoughts, and feelings are unforgivable, do not live up to their own standards, or will endanger them. The crux of the problem in self-criticism is the contempt and the harshness and hostility with which the criticisms are directed toward self. It is interesting to note that in depression the intensity of the affect associated with self-criticisms appears to be much higher than in nondepressed clients.

Interpersonally Related Determinants. Here the focus can be on current relationships or unresolved issues in past relationships:

1. *Interpersonal dependence.* Loss, or threat of rejection, disapproval, or abandonment, involves the fear of being hurt and the fear of not being able to cope or survive when needs for closeness or support are not met. For example, one client had a frantic reaction to her partner not listening to her, while another avoided intimacy for fear of being abandoned again. The goal is to access the basic insecurity and the primary fear or sadness underlying the desperation, along with the associated action tendencies and meanings. These can then be restructured by reowning, experiencing agency, and symbolizing the feeling. Saying "*I* feel shattered," "*I* feel all alone," and truly accepting this, rather than panicking, worrying about the future, or blaming the other, promotes agency. By identifying the feeling, for example, of feeling shattered, the need is more easily accessed and reowned and can then be more easily regulated. The client can then acknowledge, "I need to feel safe and protected or I need support or companionship." Self-soothing capacities can be accessed to overcome extreme dependence on others for affect and esteem regulation, or action can be mobilized to get needs met.

2. *Unresolved feelings toward a significant other.* This "unfinished business" often involves unresolved issues of intimacy and control, especially dealing with childhood maltreatment or past traumatic situations with a significant other (Greenberg et al., 1993; Paivio & Greenberg, 1995). The emotional responses continue to resurface and interfere with functioning long after the event or the relationship has changed or ended. The goal is to access incompletely processed primary emotion and express and reprocess it. This promotes self-empowerment and separation. Additionally, the goal can be to access and restructure maladaptive emotion schemes—beliefs about self and others formed at the time of trauma.

Individualized Determinants. In addition to the foregoing three classes of specific determinants, idiosyncratic determinants may become the ongoing focus for therapy. Issues such as not knowing what one wants, needing to make a decision, or feeling highly vulnerable may capture clients' core issues or predominant cognitive–affective processing problems. Our approach to formulation involves ongoing process diagnosis of current in-session problems rather than a diagnosis of the overall personality (Goldman & Greenberg, 1996, 1997). Thus we always focus on what emerges as most important for the client. There is always the need, however, to balance fluidic attunement to current processes with an understanding of the broader goals of therapy that have been collaboratively determined. For example, if it has been previously determined that the client wants to resolve painful issues with a parent, and this has not been discussed for a few sessions, the therapist might ask, "Where are you at concerning the issues with your mother?" This refocusing on themes is especially important in time-limited therapy.

Develop Awareness of Agency in Creation of Experience

Early in therapy a shift takes place from clients' reactions toward exploring client agency in the creation of their problematic experience. The realization that current experience is not inevitable but is in some fashion self-determined is at the essence of taking personal responsibility. Moving from avoiding internal experience or blaming others to exploring the nature of one's own reactions is central in developing awareness of agency in the creation of experience.

This focus on overcoming avoidance and taking responsibility for one's agency in the construction of reality occurs in a nonblaming fashion, in a context of exploring a problem. Therapists do not give a message to clients that they are responsible for their own distress, but rather a collaborative effort emerges of inquiring into *how* the client's psychological processes contribute to the distress. The message is "Let's explore what happens in you that leads to this feeling." Interventions target sequences of internal experience and meaning and client agency in these and in the construal process. This underlines how clients are creators of their own experience rather than passive victims of events and experience.

Awareness of agency fosters a sense of control over experience and a healthy detachment from certain experience. Becoming aware that one is, for example, an agent who is thinking self-critical thoughts is far different from believing the thought and being overwhelmed by its implications. Thus when clients are able to say,

"I'm aware of thinking I'm a failure," they are adopting quite a different stance to their experience than when they say, "I am a failure." Interventions such as "So you feel bad when you criticize yourself for falling short" or "So it's when you get the feeling 'I won't be able to survive' that you begin to panic" highlight sequences and client agency in the creation of their experience. The subtle emphasis on agency and personal responsibility in these interventions begins to help people to experience that they are agents in the creation of their personal realities and that, rather than being passive victims, they have some control over this.

Experimenting to explore how clients create their own experience is useful. Often framing people's functioning in terms in which they are seen as having parts or multiple voices that serve different functions is particularly effective for enhancing people's sense of themselves as creators of their own realities. It also allows enactments of how people scare themselves or punish themselves. For example, a client who was sexually abused and whose experience was minimized and invalidated by her parents had come to doubt herself, with one voice saying, "Maybe I'm making mountains out of molehills or exaggerating." At a marker of self-doubt such as "Maybe I'm making too big a deal, maybe I should just let it go," the therapist can respond, "That's what happens, it seems, when you start to speak up with one voice—you stop yourself with another. Come over here, in this chair. Try doing that some more. Make yourself feel unsure."

Helping some people become aware *that* they avoid their experience, and of *how* they avoid or interrupt their experience, helps them become aware of their agency in the avoidance. This in the long run helps them become aware of their experience. Tracking a person's problematic reactions to situations (Greenberg et al., 1993; Rice, 1984) to get at what stood out for them in those situations and how they construed these cues also helps shift the emphasis to their agency in their interpretation of reality. In addition, exploring with clients how they avoid or suppress feelings highlights their agency in these processes.

Clients can be further encouraged to become aware of agency by observing their own experience with the use of awareness homework. Clients are asked to become aware of their many voices, what they say to themselves and how they create certain states. Rather than attempting to prematurely change these states, clients are encouraged to be aware of the processes that generate the states. By observing themselves, they will gather new information and become aware of their agency in the creation of the experience. Awareness of agency in the creation of experience is a subtle but very important change process.

Provide a Rationale

Sometimes it is necessary to explicitly provide a rationale as to how working with emotion will help. When, for example, it is judged necessary to explicitly direct clients to attend to internal experience, it can be explained why such a task would be useful. The rationale is offered in individualized form, relevant to the shared understandings of the client's unique problems. The general rationale, however, is that feelings are adaptive guides to action, provide information about reactions, and need to be acknowledged and, if dysfunctional, to be modified.

PHASE II: EVOCATION AND EXPLORATION

Evoke and Arouse Bad Feelings in the Session

In order to change experience in the session the experience needs to be evoked right there (Rice, 1974). The therapist's actions in this phase are intended to be predominantly present centered to analyze current expression and to intensify experience and evoke memories. In addition, in order to maintain the alliance, there needs to be agreement about the tasks undertaken to access the bad feelings and address the difficulties. The client needs to perceive the tasks of therapy and the evocation of the bad feelings as relevant to the kinds of changes desired (Bordin, 1979; Horvath & Greenberg, 1994; Watson & Greenberg, 1994). How the troublesome feelings are activated in the session depends on the process-diagnostic assessment of the specific generating conditions. This step involves two subprocesses, evoking experience and attending to avoidance and interruption of emotional experience.

Evoking Emotional Experience

Bringing experience alive involves the use of some type of emotion stimulation. It involves attending to different features of experience. Using a network analogy, one "primes" the nodes of relevant associative networks or, in terms of levels of processing, one weights certain information in a current synthesis more highly. It does not involve linear reasoning, the identification of patterns of behavior or experience across situations, or behavioral or situational tracking. Thus the therapist moves between verbal meaning and nonverbal experience and expression, between past and present, between bodily sense and visual imagination, all in a nonlinear manner in order to prime different nodes of the emotion-generating schemes (Greenberg & Safran, 1987; Greenberg et al., 1993).

Once a client's emotion scheme has been evoked, information is accessed in a "hot" fashion. Emotional meaning is then symbolized and reflected on. This, in turn, feeds back and activates further emotion schemes or moderates the existing ones. Once the emotion scheme is "up and running" it is more amenable to change, right on the spot.

For example, a client talking about her difficulty in letting go of an unsatisfying relationship is asked how she feels when she imagines her partner. This activates an emotion scheme. She says she feels warm, likes his arms around her, feels pride, and thinks maybe they could work it out. The therapist notes that part of her really responds to and wants him, and that this makes it hard to leave. The client nods, but holds her breath and then says that she also feels smothered and claustrophobic. A second emotion scheme has been evoked. The therapist responds, "So with your longing for him, you forget, you lose sight." The client says, "Yes, but its always there, the frustration, it always come back to that. I can't do it anymore (*weeps*)." The therapist responds, "It's really sad that despite the good stuff. . . ." The client, beginning to form a new emotion scheme, exclaims, "I can't go back anymore. What about me? I need nurturing and support too. I never got it from him. I feel like he sucks me dry, there's nothing left." The therapist acknowledges, "Yeah, like it's not fair, sounds like you're not willing to sacrifice. . . ." The client reflects on her newly experienced sense of feeling depleted and says, "I am only delaying the inevitable, better to leave now."

When clients begin sessions by talking about what's been bothering them and recounting a past episode, the goal is to get in touch with that part of the story which is most alive for the person at the moment. Change will occur most effectively when the emotion scheme is accessed in the session and reflected on. Many techniques can be used to bring alive the emotional experience—empathic responding and more active interventions, indirect methods, and specifically structured experiments (Greenberg et al., 1993). Use of imagery and metaphoric language as well as empathic conjectures that move beyond the surface, closer to underlying feelings, are helpful in evoking feelings.

For example, a client who is out of touch with emotional experience may be taught to attend to bodily sensations, or a client who has a limited repertoire of emotion can be coached in adopting different postures or to imagine a specific situation or person in order to help access the associated emotion. Or the therapist can observe that as the client talks there seem to be tears behind the laughter. Or the therapist can ask, "How does it feel now, as you talk about this?"—or can respond, "That's the part that still hurts or bothers you." The alliance and safety of the therapeutic environment are crucial here. Therapists need to be comfortable with their own and others' vulnerable and often intense emotional expression. They must model acceptance of the full range of human experience.

In the case of underregulation of secondary or maladaptive emotion, the goal may be to regulate rather than further arouse the already overaroused bad feeling. Here techniques discussed in Chapter 5, such as attending to breathing regulation to reduce arousal or identifying the cognitions generating the secondary feeling, can be carried out in the session to help regulate the overaroused emotion. This helps make the primary emotion more accessible.

Attending to Avoidance and to Interruptive Processes

The complement to arousing the bad feeling is to work on becoming more aware of the blocking or interruption of emotion. Interventions explore the various ways clients block experience right in the session. These range from dissociation to simply stifling tears. Exploring and overcoming these interruptive processes constitute subgoals of therapy, and there needs to be collaboration about why it is important to do so and the means by which it will be done. By definition, facing what is dreaded can be threatening. Collaboration provides safety and minimizes the development of opposition, misalliances, or treatment impasses.

Emotionally focused interventions then aim at heightening awareness of the interruptive process. Clients can enact the process of interruption in an imaginary dialogue between both sides of the personality. For example, in two-chair dialogues, at markers of self-interruption, clients would be encouraged to enact (exaggerate) how they stop themselves from feeling, to verbalize the particular injunctions used, or to exaggerate the muscular constrictions involved in the interruption (Greenberg et al., 1993). Eventually this self-inhibition provokes a response, often a rebellion against the suppression, and the experiencing self challenges the injunctions or interruptive cognitions and bursts through the constrictions.

This technique, like all emotionally focused interventions, is designed in addition to unpack complex cognitive–affective processes. When the client and therapist are working to undo interruptive processes, some discussion of goals and a rationale may need to be provided in the form of a dialogue about desired change and the costs and benefits of interruption. The objective of the dialogue is for clients to come to understand just how they stop themselves from experiencing potentially adaptive emotions. Part of the rationale usually provided is that such an interruption happens automatically so one has no control over it. It seems important therefore to understand the way in which one suppresses a part of the self, so that the interruption is no longer so automatic and one can have some control or choice in the matter.

Clients are also helped to get past secondary emotional reactions that are blocking their more primary feelings. Although anger, anxiety, and shame have their adaptive functions, they also can obscure other feelings needed for adaptive functioning. Thus guilt or embarrassment may block expressiveness and sexual pleasure, and fear of rejection or anxiety over abandonment may interrupt assertive expression. Shame over loss of control or weakness may interrupt adaptive grieving. These secondary bad feelings are acknowledged but not intensified. Rather, the more primary unacknowledged feelings are attended to and developed. As stated in Chapter 3 on assessment of emotion, adaptive primary anger needs to be carefully distinguished from "defensive" secondary anger that covers hurt or unmet longings. Adaptive primary sadness that promotes the work of grieving must be distinguished from secondary helpless and depressive weeping that exacerbates feelings of hopelessness and victimization.

Unpack and Explore the Bad Feeling Experience

Unpacking experience and exploring it is the core of most therapy and takes place repeatedly over several sessions. The evoked bad feelings are usually learned secondary reactions made up of complex cognitive–affective sequences. The goal is to slow down and unpack the generating sequences, to differentiate feelings, and to get at underlying primary emotions and associated cognitions and needs. This unpacking and differentiating is done through empathic understanding and empathic exploration, and at times by enacting different aspects of the self.

Interventions used to explore clients' bad feeling experience always involve a balance between process-directiveness and empathic responding (Greenberg et al., 1993). Intervention is guided by ongoing attunement to client processes and subtleties of expression. In the process of exploring their experience, clients may recall concrete moments, reexperience aspects of past events, or move in and out of dialogues between parts of self or self and others. As the process evolves a client often begins to see things in a new way, realizing that a self-criticism is an old parental message, or that an automatic thought generates a bad feeling, or that a feeling of being judged by others is an attribution of one's own criticism onto them, or that a problematic reaction is based on the way one is viewing the situation (Greenberg et al., 1993).

We operate on the principle that there is more available to awareness than is currently symbolized and that exploration of the vague edges of consciousness will yield new information. Exploring then involves attempting to clearly symbolize felt meanings involved in the bad feeling experience but currently not fully in awareness and then to reflect on them. Identification of feeling and meaning is often quite problematic for many clients. They might become aware of tightness in their jaws and chests or a knot in their stomachs, but not be able to symbolize what they are feeling. They might, for example, mislabel an experience as anger when it is really anxiety or dread. Attending to and accurately symbolizing it as fear or dread is then an important first step. This requires concentration and a process of experientially searching one's internal experience until one captures what one is feeling or the meaning of an experience. It is a crucial function of the EFT clinician to help clients search and accurately label their experience. Empathic responding to their experience is one of the best ways to help clarify it and create new meaning.

PHASE III: EMOTION RESTRUCTURING

The new primary experience that emerges at this stage serves as a basis for reorganization of the self. The therapist's actions in this phase are predominantly intended to promote ownership, to symbolize experience, and to help the client establish intents.

Access Core Maladaptive Emotion Schemes and/or Primary Emotions

It is at the point of accessing primary emotions or core maladaptive emotion schemes that a major *shift* in the process occurs. The client now reorganizes and first accesses either a primary adaptive emotion or a core dysfunctional emotion scheme. Once an emotion is aroused it appears to have its own course, involving a natural rising and a falling off of intensity. Arousal also results in the activation of many new schemes, especially when attention is explicitly focused on the task of meaning creation after arousal. Thus it is the combination of arousing and symbolizing feeling that carries forward the process of meaning construction. One feeling follows another in a process that consists of the allowing, expressing, symbolizing, and completing of one emotion and the emergence of a new emotion or felt meaning. Thus fear or sadness when expressed, symbolized, and differentiated is often followed by anger; anger is followed by sadness or fear or shame; resentment, by appreciation; hate, by love; and aversion, by desire. Emergence of new feelings results in the establishment of new needs/goals. With new needs/goals, new resources are accessed to meet them. The core of the change process involves accessing primary emotional experience and directing the client's attention to emergent, alternate emotionally based needs/goals. The exploration process in Step 4 (Table 6.2) is aimed at and promotes the accessing of more primary experience. Once accessed, this serves to reorganize the person's processing. This is the emotional process that is the basis of the shift in self-organization. In this step one accesses either primary adaptive emotion or core maladaptive schemes.

Access Primary Adaptive Emotion

Previously avoided or nonsymbolized primary adaptive emotion and needs are acknowledged and experienced in this phase. As stated earlier it is not only the experience of the emotion per se but the accessing of the needs/goals/concerns and the action tendencies associated with them that are important. Thus a client, by acknowledging sadness, may experience a blocked longing to be cared for or, by newly experiencing anger, may assert boundaries. The need and action tendency associated with primary emotion leads to adaptive action. It is through the shift into primary emotion and its use as a resource that change occurs. Thus in some cases change occurs simply because the client accesses underlying anger and reorganizes to assert boundaries, accesses fear and moves away to protect the self, or accesses sadness and reorganizes to withdraw and to recover and regather resources, or reaches out for comfort and support. In these situations contacting the need and action tendency provides the motivation and direction for change. New emotion schemes are accessed or generated by this process.

In more complicated situations people contact feelings of shame or grief (sadness at loss) or deep feelings of insecurity or aloneness or pain or past trauma. These emotions need to be allowed and processed. Adaptive shame will lead to awareness of the desire to belong, grief to the grieving process, insecurity to the recognition of the need to be attached and supported, loneliness to the need to connect, and pain to the release, relief, and reorganizing process. Attending to these emerging needs/goals precipitates the reorganization, and the person begins to access internal resources to meet the goals and alternate self-views to support their attainment.

At times, this step involves explicit discussion of how to meet the newly accessed needs in the outside world and the difficulties one might encounter in these attempts. Further work on how to meet one's needs may be required. Greater awareness and acceptance of emotional experience and needs can help, in and of themselves. It is clarifying and confidence building to know what one feels, to know what are one's needs, concerns, wishes, desires, and to be able to use these as guides to action. Therapy helps people learn to trust their internal experience and to use their experience to guide them. Validation of primary experience in therapy is crucial to help people strengthen their sense of themselves and trust their experience.

Primary emotion often is accessed by verbally symbolizing feeling. This can be accompanied by a description of the physiological sensations involved in the experience of the emotion. For example, sadness might be described in terms of a heaviness in the chest, a drooping of the shoulders, and the welling up of tears in the eyes; anger, as an eruption or explosion in the chest, a clenching of the fist, and a tightening of the jaw. An exploration of the motoric action tendency may reveal, in sadness, a desire to curl up and/or be comforted; in anger, a desire to strike out. These tendencies can then be enacted in the session psychodramatically or in fantasy.

Mindless explosion or venting of emotion is not the goal; rather, experiencing the full impact of the emotion and symbolizing the emotion is encouraged until new meanings and courses of action are created. Appropriate adaptive emotional responses are generally energizing or self-soothing because they guide and protect. Thus adaptive anger involves a buildup of energy to aid in overcoming obstacles. Adaptive sadness allows for withdrawal and recuperation or reaching out for comfort that leaves one calm and able to contact the world and act.

Access the Core Dysfunctional Emotion-Schematic Network

In many instances it is complex primary *maladaptive* emotion schemes that are accessed first in therapy rather than accessing simple primary *adaptive* emotions such as sadness or anger that organize one for action and provide important information. Emotion schemes or networks, as we have said, are a synthesis of emotions, expectancies, beliefs, meanings, action tendencies, and needs (Greenberg et al., 1993). When these schemes, based on the person's emotional learning history, are maladaptive, they need to be restructured. Thus primary maladaptive feelings, such as a core sense of feeling powerless or a fear of annihilation, or feeling invisible, or a deep sense of woundedness, of shame, of insecurity, or of worthlessness, or of feeling unloved or unlovable, are accessed as the core of the evoked secondary bad feeling. Core dysfunctional experiences such as these often relate either to hostile self-criticism or to anxious dependence—in the former, to feeling worthless, a failure, and being bad; in the latter, to feeling fragile and insecure, being unable to hold together without support. These are the core bad/weak negative self-schemes. In these instances the primary maladaptive feelings of badness, weakness, or insecurity and the fears of annihilation, disintegration, and abandonment have to be accessed in order to allow for change. It is only through experience of the emotion that emotional distress can be cured.

Aided by the supportive acceptance of the therapists, what is curative is the ability to symbolize these feelings of badness or weakness and then to access alternate self-schemes based on adaptive emotions. Most people have had some "positive parenting" by someone who confirmed or soothed them in some manner and this provides a capacity for the self-affirmation, assertion, and protest as the basis of alternate self schemes. Such alternate schemes are often accessed by focusing on background or subdominant adaptive emotions that accompany the more figural maladaptive feelings. An example is focusing on the adaptive anger at violence that accompanies the traumatic fear when the trauma is recounted. The subdominant emotion is often not yet symbolized and does not yet govern the person's self-organization. Once the subdominant emotion is made figural, the person's self-organization changes and adaptive feelings and needs get activated especially in response to the currently experienced emotional distress. It is the patient's internal emotional response to their own symbolized distress, that is adaptive and must be accessed and used as a life giving resource. The steps in this process are shown in Table 6.3. In this table, we see that by focusing on subdominant emotions and/or emotional adaptive responses to the currently felt distress, life sustaining tendencies are accessed. Once these new strivings are symbolized, the self reorganizes around the newly established goals (Lewin, 1935).

Thus when a person feels bad, shameful, worthless, and rotten to the core, the associated feeling is one of sadness or shame and the need/goal is to feel acceptable and worthwhile. When one suffers the primary bad feeling of shame and worthlessness and is able to symbolize it and realize that this is what one feels (rather than avoid it), one can begin to gain some reflective mastery over it. With this realization alternate emotions and self-views and the need to feel acceptable becomes much more accessible and the person begins to feel more deserving of having the need met. Thus, one may access subdominant adaptive feelings of sadness or anger at what was missing and this helps

TABLE 6.3. The Essence of Accessing Emerging New Feelings

1. How do you access alternate primary emotions?
   Focus on subdominant emotions that have been evoked with the maladaptive emotions and on emotional responses to the evoked emotions
2. What do you do then?
   Focus on goals/motivations in newly accessed emotions that promote adaptive coping.
3. Why?
   The self-organizing system reorganizes around the new goal/motivation and challenges dysfunctional beliefs.

motivate new needs/goals/concerns and new self-organizations. This occurs especially in an empathic, validating, and supportive therapeutic environment. People are more able to be *empathic to themselves* when they are both actually experiencing their suffering and are receiving empathy from another. They simultaneously need to experience their distress and to step back sufficiently to see themselves, to empathize with themselves, and symbolize their own pain and suffering. Once they have stepped back and have a place from which to view themselves, they have already reorganized and the processing *shift* has occurred. With the added empathy and support of the therapist, clients then are able to reorganize in response to their own emerging feelings, their emotional distress, and their need. Motivated both by their aversion to pain and by their need for mastery and contact comfort, new resources are mobilized enabling them to better cope with these demands. An alternative more adaptive self-scheme is contacted or generated, and this acts as a basis for challenging or restructuring the core maladaptive scheme.

Thus a client after clearly symbolizing in awareness her feeling of worthlessness by saying, "I feel so worthless," sobbed with the full realization of that feeling. At a particular moment, acting as a dynamic system in a process of change, a new feeling emerged and she suddenly reorganized and another need/goal/concern emerged. Her sadness at missing the support she had never received now rose to the fore and replaced the shame. Once her new affectively based need/goal for survival and attachment related to her new sadness was accessed, a new self-scheme became available. She contacted an inner wellspring of self-worth and said, "I am worthwhile, I deserve to be valued" and "I have love to give, and I deserve to be loved." When people feel insecure, fragile, and unlovable and are unable to regulate their own anxiety, full experience and symbolization in the session of the feeling of being shattered, broken, desperate, or discarded can provide a sense of distance from, containment of, and mastery over the maladaptive feeling. Once people are able to say "I feel shattered" from an agentic stance, a stance that emphasizes the active "I" self rather than the shattered "me" self, they are more in charge and then are able to access new feelings, a new goal, and an alternate self-scheme. The therapist can often facilitate this reorganization, at the right time, by focusing the client on emerging feelings and needs/goals, asking such things as "What are you feeling right now?", "What do you need?", or "What has been missing?" The emerging goal now generally is no longer one of desperately needing others' approval or love to prevent being shattered. Rather, the goal has become one of supporting oneself or mastering the situation, accompanied by the agentic desire to be close, to love and be loved, or to feel safe.[1]

People, then, by acknowledging their emerging primary feelings in a therapeutic environment that both validates them and focuses them or their growth-oriented needs/goals, are able to access their organismic strengths and capacities, and these are used to construct a new self-view. At this point they feel a greater sense of entitlement to having their needs met and, no longer feeling shattered, are able to say, "Even if he doesn't respond to me, I still deserve it." They now also are able to reevaluate the consequences of their needs not being met by the other. With support from the therapist, clients therefore utilize their mastery motivation and their pain avoidance motivation to access new resources to cope with such challenges. In this way more self-enhancing and self-soothing capacities are accessed to help the person cope. The person might say, "I do deserve to feel loved. If I can't get it here, now, I can get it from within, or from somewhere else. I can survive if he doesn't respond to me. I know I won't actually fall apart."

In addition, while the feeling of worthlessness or insecurity is experienced and symbolized, the elements of the dysfunctional beliefs or expectancies, embedded in the maladaptive emotion scheme, are made accessible by the person being in the aroused state. The elements

---

[1]After a feeling of worthlessness, a fear of disappearing, or a core inadequacy or insecurity is experienced and accepted, attention must be shifted to the needs/goals. This creates new priorities. Once the feeling is symbolized and put into language, attention is focused on the need with questions such as "What do you need?" "What did you want?" or "What was missing?" What occurs in information-processing terms is that attention is shifted to focus on a new goal, generally one striving for mastery or attachment or a survival-related need. This produces a sudden reorganization (Goldstein, 1939, 1951). The need is validated and its recognition and mobilization begins a process of reorganization. The person then begins to feel entitled to the need, or begins to recognize that he or she did not previously feel so entitled and to question why this was so. This is the process the therapist attempts to facilitate.

of the state-dependent beliefs are obtained in their deepest and most essential form—in the emotional meaning context in which they operate. Now they can be articulated and conceptualized. This "hot cognition" is obtained in a truly felt manner and is not just a conceptual statement, made without any emotional investment. Thus the belief is more easily accessible to articulation and is more amenable to the input of new information and experience and thereby to change. It is the realizing that I see myself in certain ways, as articulated by the belief, that is very important. Disembedding from one's view and getting a metaperspective on how one views oneself and the world opens one up for change. The therapist does not challenge but reflects the belief, holding it up for further inspection.

In summary, in accessing core dysfunctional emotion schemes it is the emergence of newly aroused subdominant primary feelings and the mobilization of alternative, adaptive emotional needs/goals and the access to, and articulation of, the core dysfunctional expectancies and beliefs that are potentially mutative. Awareness of these enables the person to internally challenge the belief from the newly mobilized needs and resources. In addition, articulation of the belief in consciousness—speaking it out loud in the session—exposes it to reflective reevaluation and exploration.

Restructure by Promoting Articulation of and Challenges to Dysfunctional Beliefs by Adaptive Needs and Resources

As we have said, in addition to accessing the newly aroused adaptive feeling and need, the expectancy or belief associated with the emotion scheme is articulated. It is of interest to note that different patterns of beliefs and needs are generally associated with different classes of problematic experience (Guidano, 1987, 1991a, 1991b).

In this restructuring phase the clients arrive at articulations of their beliefs and at new understandings of formative experiences in their lives. Clients come to recognize and articulate the expectancies or beliefs embedded in the schemes, and also to see how their lives were structured both around these and around attempts to protect themselves against the beliefs and the associated bad feelings. Thus people vulnerable to feeling either worthless or unlovable see how much of their behavior and experience was organized to both defend against this view as well as to seek disconfirmations of this view (cf. Weiss, Sampson, & the Mount Zion Psychotherapy Research Group, 1986). Thus, clients, come to see that their felt views of "never being good enough" or "not being able to rely on anyone" govern their experience. This acknowledgement, or ability to see their way of seeing the world, gives a greater sense of understanding and control, and this awareness allows for the possibility of changing this belief. Change is essentially accomplished by disputing the belief from an awareness of how it came to be constructed and from a felt sense of alternate views of the self.

Once the dysfunctional belief, accessed via emotional arousal, has been symbolized in an emotionally rich context, it is thus challenged from within by the newly accessed and validated need/goal and by the additional resources mobilized by this need. Thus the need to be loved or recognized that is at the core of a feeling of worthlessness is accessed and supported by the therapist, and this is used to combat the belief that the person is worthless or unlovable. A person may say, "I needed support not criticism. I deserved more. I was only a child, I needed love," thereby combating beliefs about worthlessness or weakness.

The therapist supports the emergence of internal strengths, competence, and internal resources to combat negative cognitions and core maladaptive schemes. A person's internal support and self-soothing capacities also are evoked in response to the person's symbolization of distress and recognition of the core feeling and need. The sense of vitality and the will to live is contacted. People then are able to provide themselves with the support that was not obtained from others, and they begin to assert themselves and challenge self-denigrating or invalidating beliefs about the self or catastrophic assumptions concerning separation and abandonment. It is the combination of awareness of the belief, plus the therapist's support and validation, and the client's access to new needs/goals and internal resources that provides the person the strength to combat dysfunctional beliefs. In addition to the explicit challenge of newly articulated dysfunctional beliefs there is an awareness-guided restructuring process in which higher level schemes are formed integrating coactivated structures (Greenberg & Pascal Leone, 1995). Thus the core maladaptive belief governed experience of self is integrated with the newly accessed adaptive experience to form a new, stronger, more balanced sense of self.

Support and Validate Emergence of a Self-Validating Stance

Here the therapist is attuned to the emergence of clients' internal resources, self-soothing capacities, and self-affirmation. When a more confident, assertive, accepting sense of self emerges, the therapist acknowledges and validates this sense and helps the client to link this to life outside of therapy and to solve problems. The newly found sense of self-validation is used as a base for action in the world. After the client has experienced a shift in emotional process and has reorganized, the therapist and client collaborate on the kinds of actions that could consolidate the change. Frequently these possibilities emerge spontaneously. The therapist also might engage in experiential teaching to cognitively consolidate changes in perspective. Thus the therapist might underscore how, at moments of desperation, focusing internally and symbolizing one's experience to oneself—such as by saying, "I feel devastated"—helps gain a sense of mastery, or how putting oneself in the center of the experience, thereby becoming an active agent of it rather than a passive victim, helps regulate that experience. Alternatively, clients might be advised at moments of anxiety to recall their in-session experience of being more compassionate or soothing to themselves and to practice doing this. This is done only after they have succeeded in the session in overcoming their self-contempt and have become more self-supportive, so that they have this experience to draw on. Often clients report spontaneously drawing on these in-session experiences in real life.

Creation of New Meaning

The final phase of this work involves the creation and consolidation of new meaning by reflecting on what has occurred and developing a narrative of how the experience one has been through fits, or changes, one's identity. The client constructs alternative meanings and explores the implications of a new self-validating view. The goals are now to clarify an experientially based story about oneself, one's past, and one's future, and to promote actions based on the new realizations. Clients, in creating new meaning, often make connections between elements of their life, change their views of themselves or their history, and state intentions and desires to attain greater connectedness and mastery in their lives. The creation of meaning is ongoing throughout treatment and continues beyond any single emotionally laden episode of treatment, but often refers back to these episodes and to core metaphors that arose in them. Thus experientially based metaphors—such as being "alone in a vast field," "in a glass cage," "at sea in a rudderless boat," "the rising of the internal volcano," or "being thrown on a trash heap"—become symbols of problems, whereas such metaphors as "rising out of a pit" or "being able to stand firm" or "being able to freshly see again" capture emergence, development and the creation of new meanings and solutions.

Self-experience is now reorganized in such a way that the person is able to symbolize and organize emotional experience in terms of a new view of self. Thus the self is no longer judged as a failure, or separation from an attachment object is no longer perceived as dangerous to self. Both one's view of self and world and one's experience of being in the world change.

THE FRAMEWORK EXEMPLIFIED

The above process is exemplified in the following case synopsis. A 34-year-old mother of two children presents saying she is upset and that she feels like a failure as a mother because her 13-year-old daughter is in trouble. Rather than challenging this construal or getting her to collect evidence to engage in reality testing of her thoughts about whether or not she is a failure (as might a cognitive intervention) or looking for conflictual relational patterns across situations (as might a dynamically oriented intervention), EFT intervention aims at accessing and symbolizing as much internal response information as possible in order to access her primary adaptive emotional experience in relation to this problem as a guide to reorganization and action.

This is done by first exploring as concretely as possible her feelings in relation to this concern. The therapist therefore attends to and empathically acknowledges the secondary bad feeling: "I hear that you feel like you've failed as a parent and this leaves you feeling really bad inside and kind of hopeless." This helps the client feel understood and validated as a person of worth, helps her relax and bring forth more of her concrete experience, including her sinking feeling inside, the image of her daughter in trouble in the past as a young child, and her negative self-evaluations.

Once the client feels sufficiently understood and a collaborative focus has been formed to work on determining what is generating the bad feelings, her complex emotionally felt meanings related to this issue are evoked and explored to unpack the generating sequences. Thus her evoked secondary upset, hopelessness and a feeling of failure, are explored in a supportive manner. She talks about her repeated problems with her daughter, she blames herself for failing, and with the help of the therapist's empathic understanding she contacts her sense of helplessness. Exploration of this leads to even deeper feelings of powerlessness. This core maladaptive sense of powerlessness—"I can never get what I need"—learned from many life experiences, present and past, rapidly overrode her initial responses of disappointment and fear and led to her complex secondary chain of upset.

Having accessed her core maladaptive scheme of powerlessness and inadequacy, the therapist works to access the client's primary

adaptive feelings and needs/goals. Her initial primary adaptive responses to the situation, the sadness at the loss of her hopes for her
daughter and her fear for her daughter, plus her desire for her
daughter's well-being and her own needs for support, are accessed and
developed. It is the client's primary adaptive feelings of sadness and
fear and her needs/goals for mastery and attachment, at the edge of
her awareness, previously not fully attended to or symbolized, that
provide new input in the form of affectively based survival-oriented
strivings.

Thus the client, having gone into her experience of feeling inadequate and feeling hopeless, is guided by the therapist toward her
affectively based striving that had been overridden by her more figural
feelings of failure. These serve as the basis of a new self-organization.
The client, having accessed her primary sadness in the context of a
highly supportive and validating relationship, is finally able to say "I
love my daughter and I so want to help her." In this process her faulty
appraisals ("My daughter's a complete loss"), the automatic thoughts
("I'm a loser"), and the dysfunctional beliefs ("I'm a failure as a
mother") are all clearly articulated. The newly articulated views of self
are challenged from *within* by the client's newly accessed internal
resources—by her primary adaptive feelings, needs, and goals that
existed in the background as a core, essential, survival-oriented self-organization.

The client, feeling more empowered by having accessed her desire
to help her daughter, revisions her self and the situation in statements
such as "I realize I'm not a failure. My kid has good qualities as well
as bad ones. I have succeeded with my other child. It's not all my
inadequacy. I tend to go overboard on blaming myself." Thus the client,
operating from a newly formed, affectively based self-organization,
asserts that she is not a loser or failure as a mother and is able to begin
reattributing causes of her daughter's disobedience. She sees her
daughter as having succeeded in many areas but as needing some
further guidance, and the client begins to reconstrue herself as a good
mother. She now affirms herself, saying, "I do try hard. My daughter
has a rebellious and dominant personality. She'd be a handful for
anyone. It's a struggle, but I love her and she's worth it." With further
coexploration of her negative view of herself, she connects this self-
view to patterns from her past, saying, "I've always been criticized by
my parents and even my husband and I've taken it, believed it, but I
realize it's not true and I'm not going to take on that baggage any
longer."

Thus her negative cognitions have changed both by articulating
them and accessing internal affective resources to combat them. Once

her articulated, dysfunctional beliefs have been exposed, with the help of the therapist, to self-reflective evaluation, she has constructed a new narrative to explain her self and relevant aspects of her life. In addition, her sensorimotor experience, her physiological responses, memorial associations, and meaning constructions have all changed. This woman's higher level "sense" of herself has changed from feeling unworthy and hopeless to feeling worthy and hopeful.

CONCLUSION

Therapy thus involves validating clients' experience, evoking the bad feelings in the session, and exploring the emotional–cognitive sequences that generate these to get at primary emotions. If the primary experience is maladaptive, then alternate adaptive experience is accessed to restructure the maladaptive schemes. The needs/goals/concerns in adaptive emotional responses are focused on to inform action, challenge dysfunctional beliefs, and promote reorganization and access to internal resources such as self-soothing. Finally, conscious reflection, thought, and reason decide on courses of action, and they put our feelings in perspective and create new meanings.

PART THREE

DIFFERENTIAL WORK WITH THE EMOTIONS

CHAPTER SEVEN

Anger

ANGER IS A POWERFUL emotion that has a profound impact on social relations and self-organization. Anger can be stimulated by many sources. Many types of anger responses are possible—some positive, others negative, and only some aggressive. Anger is often directed at those we love for perceived wrongdoing. The typical expression of anger is intended to correct the situation or prevent its recurrence.

Anger stems from a biological tendency to defend oneself when attacked or to protect oneself from intrusion. The action tendency associated with anger involves changes in breathing and vascular, vocal, muscular, and facial responses that ready a person to thrust forward and attack the intruder. These responses organize one for action but do not actually produce behavior. The actual behavioral response results from a complex interaction of the action tendency with cognitive processes that follow the initial action disposition. The strength of the tendency to action varies, as does the subjective experience of anger, which can range from irritation, through annoyance and anger, to rage.

PROCESS DIAGNOSIS OF DIFFERENT ANGER STATES

The multileveled complexity and difficulty in differentiating among anger states is illustrated in the following example of a client in short-term therapy for depression. This client seemed chronically irritable and angry, and described herself as "getting in the shower in the morning and, by the time I'm through, I am ready to kill." Her chronic irritability needed to be explored to understand the underlying determinants. At the same time, she was annoyed with herself and felt guilty about being angry because she believed she had a good life with "everything going for me." This the therapist considered a secondary reaction-to-a-reaction that needed to be bypassed in order to access the more core experience. Finally, she expressed primary anger at years of neglect by her alcoholic mother. This was suppressed and left her complaining about and experiencing lingering resentments toward her mother. Appropriate intervention would help her acknowledge and fully express this primary adaptive anger. However, primary anger was mixed up with instrumental anger toward her mother. She stated that she realized she was holding on to her anger because it enabled her to win a kind of power struggle with her mother. It let her mother know that she was wrong, and it legitimized the client's grievances. This needed to be explored in order to understand her underlying motivations. Treatment, therefore, required different interventions at different times for the different anger states. The choice of intervention was dependent on the most salient experiential state at the moment. The following subsections describe how to recognize different anger states for the purpose of differential intervention.

We emphasize identifying and working with overcontrol of anger, as well as with rage that is secondary to hurt and shame. Whereas problems of chronic anger have received considerable attention and methods of anger control and stress management have been recommended, methods of dealing with problems of overcontrol and the psychological process involved have been inadequately described and explained in the literature.

Suppressed Primary Adaptive Anger

The first step in working with primary anger often is assessment and exploration of anger avoidance. Markers of anger interruption are in-session verbal and nonverbal behaviors that readily can be observed and identified. These include the following: collapsing into tears, helplessness, and depression, rather than expressing appropriate anger; numbing, intellectualization, and rational control of adaptive anger; minimization, that is, distancing oneself from angry feelings with trivia or jokes; diffuse and inappropriate anger; and lingering bitter resentments. In addition, people distance themselves from angry feelings by focusing externally and chronically blaming and complaining about people and situations. Blaming generally signals unresolved resentment, and complaining is a fusion of hurt, sadness, and anger that needs to be differentiated into the underlying primary emotions so that each can be expressed clearly and separately. Primary anger associated with violation or abuse has qualities of rage, disgust, contempt, or fear, whereas anger associated with unmet dependency needs or betrayal is colored with sadness at the loss. Again, in emotionally focused therapy (EFT), the treatment goal in these situations is to differentiate and clearly express each of the core emotional experiences.

In general, the goal of interventions designed to help clients express primary anger is to access the underlying network of felt meaning, help them acknowledge the unmet need, appropriately externalize blame and accountability, enhance self-empowerment, and facilitate assertive action.

Primary Maladaptive Anger

Primary anger is maladaptive when it no longer functions to protect the person from harm and violation, such as a primary angry reaction to intimacy because of prior boundary violations. Primary maladaptive anger is distinct from anger that is sequentially secondary to some other emotion or thought because it is the person's initial response to current situations. This type of anger is similar to learned fear responses that result from the automatic activation of a complex emotion structure or scheme that was formed in early attachment relationships. The treatment goal is to access the maladaptive emotion scheme, often using memory evocation techniques, so that it can be explored and restructured in therapy. This occurs through interpersonal learning with the therapist and by accessing healthy adult resources. Restructuring primary maladaptive emotion is more commonly the focus of EFT with fear and shame than it is with anger; it will be discussed in detail in later chapters.

Secondary Anger

Commonly occurring expressions of anger are reactions that are secondary to some other emotion or cognitive process. Although conscious thoughts or attributions of blame can be involved in anger activation, in our view these often are insufficient to *cause* anger activation. In many situations, already existing emotion, sensation, arousal, and stress contribute to cuing anger-related action tendencies and anger-producing thoughts. Expression of secondary anger can block the stress and pain that comes from other feelings by removing them from awareness. Anger helps release muscular tension and reduce high arousal levels associated with feelings such as fear or hurt. Thus a frightened parent may get angry at a child who runs into the street. Here this anger is secondary to fear but is due to a rapid sequence in which the parent appraises danger, feels afraid, blames the child, gets angry, and then acts to discharge the fear arousal. Similarly, a person who feels hurt when criticized or rejected can then appraise the situation as unfair and decide that the other should not have done what was done. In the same way, anger momentarily erases guilt, feelings of unworthiness, and depression: rather than feel guilty or worthless, one can blame or criticize the other; rather than feel sad, one can get angry at something or someone else to obliterate the painful sensations and thoughts.

Our therapeutic goal, in these situations, is to unpack the cognitive–affective sequences and access the more primary feeling that leads to anger. We are less concerned with modifying anger-triggering cognitions or providing coping or management skills. Our approach to secondary anger can be integrated with implicit or explicit anger-management skills training for problems of anger underregulation, but we see the ultimate goal as accessing the more helpless core emotion.

Assessing which is a core or primary emotional response in a given situation is achieved through knowledge of the activating situation, the client's learning history, and the adaptive function of primary emotion. Client verbal and nonverbal behavior, such as vocal quality, also provides important markers for moment-by-moment intervention. For example, in the initial stages of therapy, a client and therapist collaboratively agreed that her dominant emotional response was anger and that she was less in touch with other emotions. She complained as well of a fragile sense of herself, and frequently expressed fear of dissolution and abandonment. During one session, as the client spoke angrily about her partner's lack of attention, the therapist was aware of a desperate and panicky quality in her expressions of anger, and this suggested underlying fear. The therapist redirected attention to her experience of fear by tentatively reflecting the panicky quality of her voice: "It's almost as if you started feeling desperate, like it feels utterly intolerable, almost as if you can't survive without his support." Immediately her eyes welled up with tears and she acknowledged her neediness and deep fear of abandonment, which the therapist validated and accepted. The focus of therapy became unmet dependency needs, strengthening her sense of self, and looking for ways to get her needs met, rather than expression of anger.

Similarly, therapists need to both accept clients' secondary rage and work beyond it to access underlying vulnerability (Nason, 1985). It also is important to understand how an initial adaptive anger reaction can escalate into rage by a maladaptive sequence of feelings and thoughts that progressively intensifies the anger. In this sequence, every successive provocation, either a thought, perception, or interaction, becomes a new trigger for further surges of anger and each builds on the moment before. Anger builds on anger, and rage unhampered by reason easily erupts into violence. Thus, in addition to accessing and transforming helpless dependence or shame that leads to rage, it can also be helpful to unpack the cognitions that contribute to rage and to teach anger-management skills. One of these skills is learning to become aware of and express one's rising primary anger, early in the sequence, as an important means of altering the sequence.

Another common type of secondary anger takes the form of hostile self-criticism, which damages self-esteem and generates feelings of shame, failure, guilt, or depression. This form of secondary anger directed at the self can be recognized in therapy by self-contempt and self-denigration for perceived transgressions, shortcomings, flaws, unacceptable behavior, or emotional experience. Emotionally focused interventions heighten awareness of how much it hurts to be the recipient of such hostility and rejection, rather than on the anger per se. This will be dealt with in detail in Chapter 10 on shame.

Another example of anger directed at the self is a reaction-to-a-reaction, when people get angry at themselves for feeling depressed, needy, or fearful. Again, the emotionally focused therapy objective is to bypass the secondary anger at self and direct attention to the more core affective experience, the rejected part of self that feels fearful or depressed. For example, a client chastised herself for being unassertive, "childish," and "such a wimp," because she was unable to say no to others' demands or requests. The therapist assessed this anger as a secondary reaction to a more core experience of insecurity. Rather than focus on her anger, the therapist responded, "It's as if you feel like a little child and there's something very scary, very awful about others' disapproval." This was not a direct challenge but a symbolization of the intensity of her experience and need. It opened up the session to exploration of her fear of disapproval and dependency on others' approval, rather than her anger.

Instrumental Anger

Instrumental anger is a learned use of anger as a means of regulating others for secondary gains. Anger expression is an effective way to control others but usually results in them becoming bitter, resentful, and distant. Instrumental anger is frequently observed in drug rehabilitation and forensic settings, where individuals have learned to use anger to manipulate or intimidate others. This type of anger is most appropriately confronted or interpreted to foster understanding of the client's underlying motivation and aims, and teach alternative responses for achieving those aims. It is not aroused and experientially explored.

Many clients are not aware of the instrumental function of their anger, which cannot then be considered deliberate manipulation. For example, a client was hurt and angry at her parents' lack of support and reacted by "punishing them," "teaching them a lesson," "treating them the way they treat me." These are markers of instrumental anger mixed with primary anger at unmet needs. The therapist acknowledged and validated her anger at unmet needs for support but also empathically confronted her attempts to force her parents to give her what she wanted by suggesting, "It seems that no matter what you do they will never give in and all your efforts are simply pushing them further away. It's not helping you get what you so desperately want and need." This helped her let go of futile efforts to control her parents and, at the same time, supported her primary adaptive needs and motivation to achieve her goals in the world. Therapy, then, focused on finding more adaptive behavior for accomplishing these goals.

EMOTIONALLY FOCUSED INTERVENTION

We use these following elements in a sequenced and integrative manner. First, we emphasize accessing primary adaptive anger that is out of awareness. Arousal and expressive techniques can be emphasized initially in order to promote allowing of disowned anger. This is followed by acceptance and exploration of the meaning of anger, as well as awareness of the needs, demands, and expectations underlying the anger and any associated dysfunctional beliefs. Reowning primary adaptive anger and, less frequently, restructuring maladaptive emotion schemes in order to modify maladaptive primary anger are the goals. Coping approaches, on the other hand, are seen as more appropriate for dealing with secondary anger and to help control violence and rage. However, we believe that work with rage also can require accessing and acknowledging underlying vulnerability and powerlessness. This can be combined with teaching anger-control techniques and new ways to communicate in order to get needs met.

Intervention Principles Relevant to Anger

Although all of the intervention principles are applicable to therapeutic work with all of the emotions, here and in subsequent chapters (8–11) we will highlight those that are particularly important to the specific emotion considered in each chapter. The following principles are particularly relevant to work with anger.

Attending to Bodily Felt Sense

The bodily experience and action tendency associated with anger include feelings of tension, heat, pressure, energy, and power, the press for expression, the desire to "let it out," to yell, kick, pound, push the offender away, to separate, or to take a stand. Because of this explosive, outwardly directed bodily experience, active interventions are particularly powerful for helping clients express primary anger. For example, in empty-chair work (Daldrup, Beutler, Engle, & Greenberg; 1988; Greenberg & Safran, 1987; Greenberg et al., 1993; Paivio & Greenberg, 1995), the client expresses anger toward an imagined significant other in the empty chair. In directly confronting the imagined offender, clients are able to enact and say, in the safety of the therapy situation, what they have been unable to do and say in real life.

Anger can be very powerful, and therefore it is commonly over-controlled because of social injunctions against its expression, as well as fear of being overwhelmed or hurt by it. In order to engage in active expression in therapy, clients must feel assured that their anger will be accepted and contained, so that they will not hurt or embarrass themselves or others. Clients who are highly reactant or socially anxious may find it difficult to engage in the active expression of anger, and work with such clients can require the use of more responsive interventions in which the person's anger is symbolized and confirmed as valid.

When the most salient internal experience is an effort to control emerging anger experience, the therapist will direct the client to attend to that process. Attention is focused on interruptive processes as they occur moment by moment rather than a pattern of avoidance. This is illustrated by a novice therapist who, at a process marker of anger interruption, asked her client, "You shut down—what do you think makes you do that?" This led to an intellectual analysis of the client's pattern of avoidance, rather than experiential exploration of the process, moment by moment. The latter would be facilitated better by a response such as "How did you do that just now, shut yourself down? Let's explore what just happened." That sort of response specifically directs attention to the present experience.

Symbolization

Therapists can help clients by symbolizing both their anger and even more their anger interruption. They can do the latter by tentatively suggesting possible interruptive processes. For example, with the above client, the therapist might have said, "I don't know, sometimes people stop themselves by saying something like 'what's the point? Why bother being angry? You'll never get what you want anyway,' or 'Don't let her know she gets to you,' or 'Don't be angry. You'll end up like a raving lunatic.' " These suggestions are empathic guesses based on the therapist's knowledge of the client and attunement to the client's in-session process. The therapist observes whether anger interruption typically leaves the client hopeless, or controlled and tense, or whether she or he fears criticism, and so on.

Intensification of Arousal

This is one of the most difficult aspects of anger intervention for novice therapists. If they are threatened by intense anger or nervous that the client's anger will be out of control or escalate into violence, then intensification should be avoided. In deciding to use intensification strategies, therapists first need to be confident that the client's problem is one of overcontrolled primary adaptive anger and they also need to be clear about the purpose and value of intensification at any given moment.

Strategies to intensify anger experience include phrases such as "How dare you?" directed at an imagined other. This can follow analysis of expression in which clients are asked to exaggerate or repeat (e.g., "Do it again," "Say it louder") a phrase or gesture, such as pounding their fist or yelling. Such strategies also can include the use of aids, such as using a soft bat to hit a pillow, in order to heighten arousal and enable bodily cues to stimulate emotional experience. These stimulators are intended to heighten arousal and overcome overcontrol of anger when it is therapeutic to acknowledge, accept, and fully experience previously suppressed primary anger. This releases the adaptive action tendency and provides orienting information.

As well as intensifying arousal, therapists help the client to symbolize the implicit action tendency associated with their aroused anger with responses such as "Get away from me" or "So angry you'd like to beat on him." In empty-chair dialogues with an imagined other, clients can be asked directly what they would like to do and, if appropriate, encouraged to enact doing it. In cases of abuse, for example, anger experience can be intensified by encouraging clients to talk about their revenge fantasies. This can require preparatory work to educate the client about differences between experiencing and expressing rage in the safety of the therapy session and acting on it elsewhere. In general, clients are not encouraged to enact destroying the other. Importantly, the therapist guides physical expressions so they are deliberate and used in conjunction with symbolization of specific injuries or offenses, such as "I'm angry at you for beating on Mom" or "How dare you use me and humiliate me."

The above interventions are in obvious contrast to anger-management strategies intended to dampen arousal. They are contraindicated for problems with underregulated or out of control secondary anger. Active expression can be balanced with management skills and teaching the clients to differentiate their anger states. Particular cautions are necessary when clients are dealing with suppressed rage. Revenge fantasies, for example, are understood as an expression of how much the person has been injured. Such desires to hurt the other are normalized as indicators of the extent of the damage to self, a sign of unresolved anger, a desire to hurt the other the way one has been hurt. Clients can be encouraged to say things such as "I'm so furious I'd *like* to. . . ." This type of expression is only one phase in the process and appropriate only with clients who have sufficient ego strength not to become disorganized or be overwhelmed by intense emotions, who are clear about the difference between expression in the safety of the therapeutic situation and acting out, and who are not at risk for violence or self-harm.

There are individual differences in expressive style, and the degree of intensity always depends on the individual and the situation. Unproductive interventions that intensify anger expression without promoting authentic experience are little more than enactments "full of sound and fury signifying nothing." Therapists need to be clear on the purpose of intensifying anger experience. It accesses emotion, aids in completing the emotion cycle, and heightens awareness of unmet needs, thereby promoting self-assertion, self-empowerment, and separation. It also teaches clients to accept and tolerate their anger and work with it rather than against it.

Promoting Ownership and Agency

Although anger is experienced and expressed with an external focus, the type of anger expression encouraged in therapy is not blaming and hurling of insults at others but involves a movement toward greater assertive expression. The focus is on awareness of internal experience and the promotion of ownership and agency by encouraging speaking from the internal experience. Responses such as "It sounds like you're angry at not having your efforts at least acknowledged," which include a focus on the implicit wants, needs, and expectations associated with anger, help clients attend to and express their own concerns rather than blame the other. In empty-chair work, a client who feels victimized and says, "You used me," might be encouraged by this suggestion: "Try saying, 'I resent (or hate) what you did.' " In imagery, one is asked to experientially enter the image, to identify with and speak from the self, rather than to intellectually analyze the image.

However, when the client's problem is maladaptive self-blame or guilt, an important aspect of anger expression involves the appropriate externalization of blame. This is commonly the case with clients who have been abused. Expressions of anger that externalize blame and come from a legitimate and deep sense of violation and injustice need to be encouraged. These feelings are powerfully assertive and focused, and involve holding the other accountable rather than simply hurling insults. They have the effect of empowering the client rather than reinforcing a victim stance (Greenberg et al., 1993; Paivio & Greenberg, 1995; Paivio et al., 1996).

THERAPEUTIC WORK WITH PRIMARY ANGER

In general, EFT with both anger and sadness involves accessing the primary adaptive emotion in order to access the adaptive action tendencies. We have organized the examples of working with primary anger in terms of five different affective tasks that illustrate different intervention strategies: (1) overcoming rational overcontrol and unassertiveness; (2) resolving lingering resentments and bad feelings; (3) resolving anger due to betrayal or abandonment; (4) expressing anger at trauma and abuse, and (5) focusing of chronic anger. In describing these episodes, and the episodes in the chapters that follow, we are not intending to offer case formulations but to offer descriptions of emotion processes in specific contexts, in order to spell out the relevance of these processes to overall treatment and outcome. In each of the following episodes we will highlight the eight intervention steps of EFT outlined in Chapter 6. The examples that follow often use empty-chair dialogue to promote the expression of anger. Although this is a useful method, we do not mean to suggest that this is always the best or the only way to work with anger. It is the process of accessing experiencing and expressing the anger that is important, and this can be done in any way that facilitates it.

Rational Overcontrol and Nonassertiveness

The two major psychological problems that occur with anger are its overcontrol and its overactivation, with associated problems of under-regulation. These problems are not mutually exclusive, as illustrated by the "bottle-up–blow-up syndrome," in which the chronic overcontrol of anger leads to inappropriate and explosive anger. Suppressing anger to even small degrees in situations that are perceived as attacks prevents assertive action. This, then, exacerbates a feeling of weakness and disempowerment, which engenders more anger. Spiraling sequences of this sort leave people feeling "full of anger" and result in an exaggerated, explosive, and ineffective expression of anger.

The automatic overcontrol of anger is as important a psychological problem as chronic undercontrolled anger and instrumental anger used to dominate or control. People often suppress their adaptive angry reactions at being violated or hurt; in such situations of overcontrol, control and management strategies are inappropriate. When anger is chronically overcontrolled, problems become infinitely more difficult to recognize and resolve. In these situations, people are unable to assert their boundaries or defend themselves from attack or harm and primary adaptive anger needs to be acknowledged and expressed, rather than managed or controlled.

One of the potentially destructive consequences of holding in anger is that individuals also are avoiding making clear statements about what they need, want, and think. Thus interpersonal problems commonly associated with anger avoidance are lack of assertion and boundary definition. In addition, individuals who suppress their anger begin to lose touch with what is important to them and to feel alienated from their own needs and wants. They relinquish responsibility for their own growth and for ensuring the quality of their own lives. A major intrapersonal problem, along with alienation from self, is that avoidance of anger leaves people feeling more acutely helpless. This can be the case for those who suppress anger at having been victimized, violated, or abused.

People also experience physiological stress from expressive overcontrol. Stress results from tightening the jaw and musculature, increased heart rate, holding the breath, and stifling the shout. The constriction of angry feelings has been associated with a variety of health problems such as stomach ulcers, high blood pressure, tension headaches or migraines, and other more severe psychosomatic reactions.

Clients chronically interrupt experiences of primary anger because of social injunctions against its expression. The experience of anger can be threatening because it signals potential disapproval, rejection, or loss of a needed relationship. Thus, many women (as well as men) have learned to be submissive, unassertive, and deferential to others, thereby suppressing their own needs and swallowing their anger. Such chronic suppression can lead to depression and apathy. Having given up hope of ever getting their needs met, people lose touch with the assertive feelings, wants, and needs that define the self. The following case example illustrates EFT work with such a client.

Overcoming Rational Overcontrol

A middle-aged artist sought therapy for chronic depression, feelings of alienation, and discontent in his marriage. He complained of feeling flat, numb, and emotionally dead. This man had grown up with a violent alcoholic father and recalled, as an adolescent, wanting to kill his father, but instead withdrawing into his room, collapsing into hopelessness and helplessness. Like many clients who have grown up in dangerous or oppressive environments, he learned to protect himself by shutting down feelings, and he feared lashing out and hurting others with his anger. Currently, in his marriage, he was hurt and angered by his wife's infidelity but felt that there was no space for him to express his feelings in the relationship. Keeping tight control over his feelings was assessed as an underlying *determinant* of his bad feelings, creating tension, sapping him of energy, leaving him lifeless, disoriented, and out of touch with his needs.

Unlike the approach with the anger of the female clients described earlier, a part of this therapy involved a kind of emotion awareness training to help the client overcome emotional numbness. When asked how he felt, his typical response was "Dunno," so therapy began with directives to attend to bodily sensations, such as "What are you aware of right now as you speak about this? Go inside your body. What do you feel?" One difficulty he experienced in doing this was his limited vocabulary for emotion words, his struggle to find the perfect word, and his resultant performance anxiety. Important aspects of intervention were provision of safety and reassurance that there was no perfect word, explicit teaching in experiential search skills, as well as empathic responding, rather than asking questions about how he felt. Empathic responses directed attention to his internal experience and helped him accurately label it. This helped him feel less anxious and enabled him to let go, somewhat, of rational overcontrol so he could explore his internal experience and *access adaptive emotional experience,* including anger.

He often was aware of tension in his gut, and the therapist encouraged him to *explore* and symbolize this bodily felt sense by saying, "Stay with that tension, squeezing tight, keeping tight control on what?" This client was a painter, and the therapist used his art to help him symbolize his internal experience.

T: Go inside. What are you aware of?

C: Oh, I don't know, (*pause*) a feeling of emptiness.

T: Where do you feel that? (C: *Puts hand on chest.*) What shape is it?

C: (*pause*) It's egg shaped.

T: Stay with that, stay inside your egg. What's it like in there? Are there images or colors?.

It was important to keep him grounded in his bodily experience when he drifted into intellectual description of the organization, hues, symbolic meaning of the colors. The therapist encouraged him: "Stay in your body. Speak from that frame of reference. What is that grey-blue color saying: 'I'm sad?' " When the client replied, "No, it's a big blanket on my feelings, (*pause*) but underneath I think I'm angry," they explored what he was angry about.

Other interventions involved analyzing expressive gestures. Whenever he talked about upsetting situations, his voice was flat and his body slumped, but he tapped his hand on the side of the chair. After observing this for several sessions, the therapist finally directed him to do this some more and put words to it. She offered suggestions—"What is it, 'discomfort,' 'impatience,' 'irritability'? "—which again accessed anger, fear of anger, and attempts to control it. Thus in addition to exploring the meaning of this anxiety about anger expression, therapist responses repeatedly directed the client's attention to his primary experience and intensified it. Such increased awareness and provision of safety enabled him to acknowledge and express his anger in the session, and he began to assert his needs in his current relationships.

Lingering Resentments from Unexpressed Anger

Some clients acknowledge anger at perceived injustices and unmet needs, but chronically suppress it so that their resentments build up. Such unexpressed anger lingers on in the form of psychological and physiological discomfort, and it raises the person's threshold for getting angry about other things. Thus, individuals who refrain from clearly expressing their anger, in a direct manner and toward appropriate objects, may resort to indirect ways of expressing their anger, for example, through sarcasm or passive–aggressive behaviors.

Unexpressed anger is particularly troublesome when it accumulates over time in relationships with significant others and concerns unmet needs for trust, autonomy, competence, identity, and intimacy. The unexpressed anger and unmet needs remain as unfinished business that is reactivated by current situations that remind the person of the past unfinished event. When such unfinished business is evoked, the previously interrupted action tendency strives for completion and, as a consequence, intrudes upon the current event (Daldrup et al., 1988).

However, its expression in the immediate situation is likely to be indirect and unproductive because the reevoked anger is appropriate to a past event rather than the current one. For example, a woman who is burdened with unresolved feelings of anger toward her overbearing and domineering father can quickly become angry and uncooperative whenever people in authority, such as a boss, attempt to curtail or limit her activities.

Angry feelings such as these, which were originally blocked or inhibited, were therefore prevented from undergoing the further differentiation and refinement that are required for directing effective action. Thus, unresolved anger frequently is associated with unexpressed hurt and sadness. Resolution of such unfinished-business issues involves differentiating and clearly expressing these distinct emotional experiences with their distinct action tendencies and needs. In therapy, clear expressions of primary anger often will shift spontaneously into primary sadness or vice versa. The sadness that follows full expression of primary anger is not collapsing into victimization and tears but adaptive acknowledgement of loss. The emotionally focused therapist is responsive to the evolving moment-by-moment process and directs attention to anger when it is most alive and a core generating condition of client current bad feelings.

Client Example

A middle-aged man sought out therapy for stress and emotional conflict over having to care for his aging and senile father, whom he hated. He experienced chronic anger and impatience toward his father, was irritable and impatient with his own sons, and feared that he was reenacting the way his father had treated him as a boy. The client and therapist agreed that lingering resentments from the past were the underlying determinants of his current bad feelings and issues with his family.

Therapy sessions initially were filled with blame and complaints about the father's inconsiderate and annoying behavior. Therapy aimed at helping him shift from this external perspective and attend to and speak from his internal experience. The therapist provided the *rationale* for this shift in focus by empathizing with the client's feeling that he was stuck, that nothing ever changed with his father, that he was "spinning his wheels." She suggested that he could get unstuck by speaking from his gut, rather than spinning around on the surface of things. The therapist requested his permission to refocus his attention on internal experience whenever he deflected into external descriptions and stories. The objective was to differentiate and clearly express his feelings toward his father in order to access new and adaptive information.

Interventions included evocation of memories of numerous childhood experiences when he felt slighted, dismissed, and betrayed by his father. The therapist directed him to attend to his internal experience of hurt and anger while he explored these core memories and to explicitly tell his imagined father, in the empty chair, what he resented. This accessed primary experience of anger and unmet needs. For example, he recalled waiting for hours one Sunday for his father to play catch with him, while his father sat in the television room drinking beer and laughing with his buddies. The client was able to clearly express his feelings and say, "I resent you making me wait like that," "How dare you make me wait, be so inconsiderate," "I resent that your drinking buddies came before me," "I'm angry at you for all those times. I deserved a father who took an interest in me." He also expressed resentment about his father's inconsiderate treatment, over the years, of his mother and other family members. In this instance it was important for the client to imagine his father in the chair as much younger because he felt inhibited expressing these things to his frail old father.

As in most situations involving attachment relationships, expressing lingering resentments also accessed this client's deep hurt at his father's lack of attention. During one session, after saying how angry he felt, the client said, "I wanted so much to please you," and wept that he never succeeded and never once got a hug from his father. He was able to express to his imagined father that this is what he needed. Moreover, he recognized that even as an adult he still wanted a "pat on the head" from his father and that this is what his anger and irritability were about. Accessing this unmet need for approval and attention and recognizing his father's neglect as having more to do with his father's deficiencies than his own helped him *restructure* his view of himself and his relationship with his father. He softened toward his father, became more tolerant of his frailties and limitations as an old man, and *affirmed* his own worth, thereby resolving his unfinished business (Greenberg et al., 1993).

Anger at Abandonment and Betrayal

Anger in response to betrayal and abandonment often is mixed with sadness and, sometimes, fear and devastation. Issues of betrayal and abandonment involve not only deep hurt and feelings of vulnerability from sudden loss of support but shattered trust and damage to self-esteem. The victim perceives him- or herself as having been let down, wronged, shafted, getting a "bum deal," or cast aside, unlovable, undesirable, and rejected. The other has not lived up to obligations, responsibilities, or expectations; promises have been broken. Anger due to betrayal or abandonment partly stems from frustration at lack of control over the situation, as well as primary anger at perceived injustice, wrongdoing, uncaring damage to self, and unmet needs. Thus, work with betrayal and abandonment can be a process of facilitating normal grieving in which anger plays a more central role. As in other situations of loss, it is important in therapy to differentiate feelings of anger, hurt, fear, and sadness. This is illustrated in the example of betrayal when one partner in a couple has had an affair. The one who feels betrayed may fear experiencing the depths of the devastation, or distrust of the offender, so is unable to express the pain. The betrayed party does not trust that he or she will be heard, understood, and protected. Shattered trust and deep lingering resentments can be indirectly expressed through distancing, coolness, and lack of connection, or steely unforgiveness and unconscious or deliberate attempts to "punish" the guilty party. One of the things that is needed for healing to take place is for the betrayed party to express the depths and intensity of his or her feelings, particularly anger, and to hold the other accountable. Then, the betrayer needs to hear, accept, and take responsibility for the pain and devastation caused, and desire to make amends. In this way the person who feels betrayed can let go, forgive at a deep level, and move on to other concerns.

A similar process seems to be necessary for healing to take place in other instances of betrayal. The victims need to believe that the offending parties would hear them, take responsibility, and seek to make amends if they could. The victim then can soften and begin to empathize with the others' limitations. This process of resolution is distinct from some situations of abuse in which resolution takes the form of externalizing blame and holding the other responsible for harm, without necessarily forgiving or understanding the other (Paivio, 1995).

Client Example

A client had suffered from symptoms of chronic posttraumatic stress since the suicide of her mother when she was 10 years old. She had been traumatized by finding her just moments after she had shot herself, and the trauma continued through the chaos and devastation that followed. She had been unable to come to terms with her mother's death, could not talk about it without shortness of breath and her eyes welling up with tears. She was deeply ashamed of her past, avoided telling others about it, experienced intrusive memories especially at anniversaries, and felt a deep insecurity. Furthermore, the chronic anger she felt at having been traumatized and saddled with this burden had been invalidated. She had been told all her life to bury the past, that there was no point in being angry because her mother was sick, and to just get on with her life. However, she viewed her mother as unforgivably selfish and abandoning and could not forgive her.

One of the aims of treatment was to validate and allow her to express her anger, because she identified invalidated anger and lingering bitterness as most troubling to her. This was seen as a first step and an integral part of grieving the loss of her mother. Empty-chair dialogue was the primary intervention, and this entailed gradual exposure to the painful *core memories* that were evoked when imagining her mother in the empty chair. The therapist coached her in regulated breathing, helped her set her own pace, and monitored her coping, both within and between sessions. (This will be elaborated on in Chapter 9 on fear and anxiety.) She was able to tolerate the dialogues and seemed to find it important to "talk" to her mother. The process helped *evoke and explore* all her feelings about this trauma in order to clarify and symbolize all the things she was angry about, so she could let go. The following is an excerpt from Session 6, in which the client is talking to her imagined mother.

EXPLORE BAD FEELINGS

C: I want you to think about those things and think about the people that you hurt by doing what you did. And the devastation. . . .

T: Can you tell her about some of those things? It sounds important. [Symbolize]

C: It's, it's very important. If you hated my father and didn't want to live with my father, why didn't you leave? I don't know if you were able to see his pain after you did what you did, but . . . you can't imagine how you hurt him. . . . You killed him as well. He died the day that you died. . . . It was easy for you because you walked away from it.

T: Mm-humm. You just walked away, you had it easy.

C: You just left it . . . like a spoiled brat. . . . Screw the world, I'm going to do what I choose to do.

EVOKE PRIMARY ANGER

T: Mm-humm. A spoiled brat. Sounds like you feel pretty contemptuous toward what she did. [Symbolize]

C: I, I do feel contempt. I never realized that . . . a great deal of contempt for what you did. . . . I blame you for not providing us with what we needed. What kind of a mother would leave three little kids?

T: It's like, I'm very angry at you for leaving us without a mother. [Symbolize]

C: Oh, yes, very, very angry at you. I was a child, and I deserved to have a mother that would give me the things that I needed until at least I got to an age where I could be self-sufficient, not to be put in the self-sufficient role at ten and a half years old.

T: Tell her again—I needed a mother, I needed care. [Establish need]

C: I needed a mother. Oh, I needed it. I needed it.

(*The therapist directs the client to switch chairs and enact her mother's response to this expression of need. The client enacts the mother asking for forgiveness.*)

T: Come over here (*directs client to switch to "self" chair*). How do you respond to her saying, "I need you to forgive me"?

C: (*pause*) I want to forgive you. It's important that I forgive you so that I can let you go, so that you can rest and I can rest. It's an important area to truly forgive you, but I'm finding it hard to forgive you in my heart. . . . It still bothers me inside. And I'm not going to reach in there, and I don't know how to reach in there.

VALIDATE SELF-AFFIRMATION

T: So still, and at that level, I'm still angry at you. I don't know how to do it yet, but I want to. [Establish intentions]

C: I want to. I want to very much.

T: Can we end for now and say we'll come back, do some more? How are you feeling about the work we did today?

The therapist *acknowledged* and understood her inability to forgive her mother and *validated* the enormity of the burden that had been thrust on her at such an early age, and her right to be angry. At the same time she highlighted the client's desire to forgive her mother. In other sessions, interventions that intensified emotional arousal, such as "Tell her how furious you are . . . say it again," were important in order to overcome avoidance of painful experience, *access* her primary anger, and facilitate its full expression. Speaking to her dead mother the client said, "I'm so angry I could throttle you," and then laughed at the irony of this. The therapist laughed with her and encouraged her to continue, "But this is how you feel." This was validating and an important part of helping her to accept her primary anger and the associated unmet needs. At the end of therapy she portrayed her mother as deeply regretful, taking full responsibility for the pain and devastation she had caused, "If there was any way I could undo it . . . ," and asking for forgiveness. This enabled the client to let go of her anger, move through the grieving process, and finally come to terms with her mother's death.

Anger from Violation and Abuse

Unresolved situations involving trauma and abuse typically are characterized by attempts to avoid painful memories of the situation. Such avoidance was originally self-protective because the person was unable to change the hostile environment, had not learned other coping strategies, or had no support for feeling the pain. Clients dealing with trauma and abuse, who suppress their primary anger, can fear being overwhelmed or losing control and hurting themselves or others. These clients need to become aware of the difference between destructive acting out, on the one hand, and the experience and expression of primary anger in the safety of the therapy situation, on the other. We believe that contained expression of primary anger, in treatment, can protect against inappropriate acting out.

Thus, therapists validate clients' rage, helping them to accept this part of their experience and allow it to run its course through active expression. Importantly, the therapy environment needs to make provision for the client's physical safety while they express intense rage. Feelings of anger may activate other emotions, such as intense fear and shame, which also require comfort and safety. The following transcript illustrates work with the effects of early trauma and fear of anger expression.

C: Perhaps, ah, it's . . . I, I feel maybe, maybe, the, the trauma began before I knew how to speak, so it makes it difficult for me to express it today? Because, ah, I can't remember not ever being afraid of my father. . . . I don't know, I just feel I've always been afraid of him, so I don't know how else to feel (T: Yeah.) and that perhaps has been a big block or a barrier to getting angry. (T: Right.) Also, uhm, just seeing my dad angry all the time and being out of control with the anger, being enraged, and out of control, I must have learned that it was bad to get angry and it wasn't . . . I would lose control if I ever (T: Yes.) got angry like him, (T: Yes.) so don't do it.

T: So there are really two aspects to it and, yes, would you be willing to try working with it?

C: Oh, yeah, yeah.

T: Ok. I do appreciate that it is difficult, but let's see how far we can take (C: Mm-humm.) this. Imagine your father over there, see what comes up. (*long pause*) Breathe again. Does that, what does that feel like? What happens to you? [Promote self-control, Direct attention]

C: (*long pause*) I . . . I want to be angry at him. But, ah, just . . . just, one look in his eyes makes me so scared. Afraid. Ah, that I can't talk, I can't say anything, I'm paralyzed to speak. (T: Hmm.) And, ah . . . (*pause*)

T: So you just can't . . . Speechless. That look, what does it do to you? Keep breathing. What . . . [Promote self-control, Attend]

C: (*pause*) It, it just paralyzes me and I just can't . . . I want to run away, but I can't run, because I can't move. I want to scream but I can't, I have no voice to scream. And the only thing that I . . . imagine that I can do is try to disappear. And, ah, pretend to hide, disappear.

T: Hmm. So you just kind of hold your breath and . . . wish for the moment to go by as quickly as possible and . . . (C: Mm-humm.) So this is how you've handled your anger, but *now*, keep breathing, in here, in this room where you don't have to confront him physically . . . can you begin to express some of these feelings. Because you don't have to make yourself disappear now. How does that feel? . . . What are you feeling? [Promote agency]

C: Right. I want to be angry at him (T: Hmm.) because maybe then I'd stop being afraid of him, but I can't find a way. I can't seem to figure out how to be angry.

EXPLORE INTERRUPTIVE PROCESS

T: Uh-huh. You don't even know where to start. I mean, there's so much it seems that you should be angry about, that you don't know where to begin or . . . is that what it's like? [Symbolize]

C: Uhm . . . Every time I think about getting angry, I just seem to . . . get very uncertain about everything. And I, I have a hard time focusing on my thoughts and, ah, I have a hard time remembering where I am in a thought, and I . . . I start doubting myself. . . . And I . . . I guess I start thinking I don't have any right to be angry and that would be wrong.

T: Hmm. Ok. So this is an important piece you know, so I'm going to ask you if you would come here and be the part of *yourself* which makes you feel like you're not entitled to this anger. Shut down, disappear or something would happen if you express it. Can you come here? (*directs client to switch chairs*) [Promote ownership and agency]

Thus, the first step in accessing anger about trauma and abuse often is to explore the interruptive process in order to restructure maladaptive fears about anger experience and expression. In the initial stages of therapy clients often find it less threatening to express anger toward a nonabusive other, such as a nonprotective parent, and this can act to desensitize fears of anger expression toward the perpetrator (Paivio et al., 1996). Eventually, however, primary anger directed toward an abusive other is important because it is associated with holding the other responsible and externalizing blame, both of which counteract internalized guilt.

Common symptoms among clients who have been repeatedly victimized are unexpressed overcontrolled rage alternating with out-of-control anger. Intervention strategies, in these cases, need to include techniques for self-soothing, anger management, and when necessary, as in the above example, decreasing arousal when the client is feeling overly anxious and panicky in the session. These are employed in conjunction with techniques to explore and unpack secondary anger that masks fear, for example, and to promote contained expression of primary anger that has been overcontrolled. Moment-by-moment assessment of the client's affective state as a guide to appropriate intervention is a critical therapy issue. EFT clinicians are attuned to "markers" of helplessness and fear underlying reactive anger and use these as signals to bypass anger and refocus on more core experience.

Again, we have found empty-chair dialogue to be a particularly effective intervention for accessing emotion memories and suppressed primary anger at trauma and violation. However, less active interventions can be used when clients find imagined contact with the perpetrator to be too aversive, provided that they incorporate the basic intervention principles. These include directing attention to internal experience, memory evocation through the use of imagery and evocative language to bring the traumatic situation alive in the session, symbolization of meaning, and establishing wants and needs as direction for future self-care.

Client Example

A man sought therapy for relationship problems with his current partner. He chronically felt distrustful, as if he was being manipulated, and would fly into fits of anger. He believed his current feelings and reactions stemmed from having been sexually molested as an adolescent, over a period of 2 years, by one of his teachers. As an adult, he had taken action to resolve the childhood abuse issue by writing letters to the local school board and newspaper. Although the client felt empowered and validated that the teacher had been released from his duties and was undergoing treatment, the issue remained emotionally unfinished. He had not fully expressed his rage and indignation about the abuse and also had never expressed his disappointment and anger at his parents, particularly his father, for not protecting him. (This aspect will be discussed in Chapter 8 on sadness and distress.) He still complained bitterly about the teacher, but in a highly intellectual, controlled, and externalized way. Thus, helping him fully express his unresolved feelings of anger and betrayal became the *focus* of therapy.

He found it difficult to engage in an empty-chair dialogue with the teacher, deflected from internal experience and from confronting the teacher directly, preferring to blame and accuse in the third person with the therapist. Thus therapy initially entailed helping him to manage his anxiety about emotional expression, as well as experiential awareness training to help him focus his attention internally, *explore his bad feelings*, and speak from that frame of reference. This was accomplished partly through structured "focusing" exercises that helped him attend to and symbolize his bodily felt sense.

Another important aspect of therapy was that his anger and disgust were mixed up with guilt and shame about his own sexual curiosity, at the time, and having responded sexually. These were pathogenic beliefs that most effectively could be explored and restructured in the process of expressing anger at control and violation, rather than challenging them at a strictly cognitive level. This was something he had done countless times already, in attempts to "talk himself out of" feeling guilty. The therapist empathically affirmed his difficulty talking about his feelings of shame and feeling tainted, as a boy, by this big dirty secret. This *accessed primary* adaptive anger at the teacher for shaming him and causing him pain.

After several sessions, he was able to relax, relinquish some control, and deeply experience and speak from his anger. With support and *validation by the therapist* he spoke of revenge fantasies, of what he would like to say and do if he met the teacher on the street, and the therapist encouraged him to imagine the teacher and express these fantasies. She also used interventions, such as "Say it again" and "Say it louder," to intensify his experience, *express* his primary anger to completion, and symbolize its meaning in terms of manipulation, victimization, and betrayal of trust. In the following excerpt, the therapist is encouraging the client to confront the imagined abuser in the empty chair.

ACKNOWLEDGE AND DIFFERENTIATE BAD FEELINGS

C: I feel so robbed, so used, but what can I do? It . . . (*sigh*)

T: Uh-huh, sort of, there's no way I can undo it all. [Symbolize]

C: Hopeless, sad.

T: Uh-huh, sad.

C: And I feel so angry at all the crap he fed me. He was such a bastard, (*looks at empty chair*) the crap you told me.

T: Right, tell him more—that's totally, that was such crap! You're so angry with him, what would you like to tell him? [Intensify]

C: Yeah, I, he is, he's, he's totally crap, nothing but trash! . . . Trash, that's all you do, you go around and you trash humanity. And what responsibilities there are, you take none of them.

T: Right, I'm furious with you for that, for not taking any responsibility, tell him how furious you are, what makes you so mad. [Promote agency, Symbolize]

EVOKE PRIMARY ANGER

C: I would really like to confront him now. . . . I would *like* him to be, sit right here in person, in front of me. Uhm, I mean I, I wouldn't, uhm . . . uh . . . you know at this point I feel, that, uhm, that I could easily confront him. . . . I think that would be kind of a final resolution, to sit him in front of me, and, and . . .. uh, work this out.

T: What would you like to say to him? . . . (C: *Expels breath.*) . . . Imagine confronting him. . . . What kinds of things would you like to confront him with? . . . (*pause*) . . .

C: . . . (*long pause*) . . . Well, I mean I, I would first just start out with impressions of him. I mean, I, he's, he's an incredible, hypocrite. *Insect!* How he can, you know, wake up in the morning, and you know, see his face in the mirror shaving, and, and, and *not* just be revolted, by himself.

T: Uh-huh, you just feel that he should be totally disgusted with himself. [Symbolize]

C: He is *so* two-faced, and he's such a creepy little hypocrite. Uhm . . .

T: What would *he* say to you? What do you imagine he'd say to your accusations and fury?

C: Uh . . . (*pause*) . . . I, uhm . . . Well, he'd try to blame it on me. He'd try to turn it back on he'd say . . . Well you, you wanted to do it all the time. And you know, you wanted to have sex with *me*. And you, you know, what do you mean calling me a hypocrite? Ta-da-da-ta-da. And you know, and that kind of thing, you wanted to do it.

T: Uh-huh. So how do you feel, thinking about that? Say, imagine that you're actually, he's here. [Focus on present, Direct attention]

RESTRUCTURE

C: You know, I think . . . How can you expect a kid, to . . . ah, adolescents are very interested in sex, and . . . this is, this is true in cases of molestation, and cases in which there is no molestation. It's just true that most young males are curious about sex, and *you played* on that. It was your fault. You had me, you know, you had the power. You had the judgment, you had the, uhm, ability to, to . . . (T: Act.) Yeah, act, (T: Properly.) responsibly. You had the choice, and you chose to, uh, *abuse,* my uh, curiosity, to . . . use my curiosity against me.

T: Say that again. It's your fault, and that I'm not to blame. [Promote agency]

C: Well it ... It was his fault. And, uh ... he knew, he'd also say something like, you know—Oh, you know, he'd try to put me down by saying ... And I would say, you know, you're a practicing hypocrite. You know, you're a little child molester, yet you put on a facade that you're *not*. You're a *total* hypocrite. And ...

EVOKE PRIMARY ANGER

T: So it's his hypocrisy that gets to you.... Stay with that, say some more. [Intensify]

C: Well! ... It drives me crazy. I trusted him, my parents trusted him, and he pretends to be so upstanding and meanwhile he's diddling little boys. He's just a low-life puke! ...

T: Yes, its important to tell him exactly how you feel, how angry you are. I feel so angry I could ... [Promote agency, Intensify]

C: Yeah, (*laughs*) I feel so angry I could...

T: Stay with your anger, what could you do to him with your anger? Its important to say. What do you feel like doing?

C: Well, yeah. I can *definitely* deal with you today. And, you know, if things escalated, I mean I would be the one that, that would start the physical violence. And I would be jailed for it undoubtedly. But, uhm, uh, uh ... you know, there's ... It would be wonderful kicking him around. Just wonderful.

T: Stay with that, you don't have to worry, it's not reality, it's what you *feel* like—I want to kick him, I'm so angry.

C: (*kicks at the chair*) I could just do this!

Therapist validation of the client's anger and desire for revenge was crucial in helping him acknowledge and express his primary experience. Once the action tendency to stand up for himself and hold the teacher accountable was released, he also was able to weep for his lost innocence. He did not forgive the teacher but *restructured* his view, seeing him now as pathetic rather than malignant, and he felt more empowered himself. At the end of treatment, he reported fewer problems with his partner, greater *self-affirmation*, and overall reduced symptom distress.

Chronic Anger

Although suppression of anger is problematic, chronic anger and a hostile outlook also cause major interpersonal and psychological problems. Anger results in elevated levels of blood testosterone in men, and epinephrine, norepinephrine, and cortisol in both genders. Chronic anger contributes to the development of a variety of diseases, including hypertension, coronary disease, and digestive disorders. Chronic anger that feeds upon itself is bad for people, whether it is expressed or suppressed, keeping them in states of hyperarousal without release. Anger also frightens others, and the angry person is experienced as dangerous. At first anger may get others to comply, but gradually others become oppositional. A sense of helplessness can underlie this chronic anger: "Unless I get angry people don't listen to me or nurture me." The anger, however, perpetuates the problem and often results in isolation and loneliness.

Chronic irritability is one of the symptoms of depression and a variety of interpersonal problems. Clients who are chronically angry seem to see offense or violation everywhere, and their expressions of anger are inappropriate and generalized. In some situations this type of anger can be viewed as a secondary reaction to more primary and vulnerable emotional experience. However, sometimes the underlying generating condition is incompletely expressed primary anger toward a specific significant other for particular harmful offenses. This is like a wound that has not healed and is continually being reopened or irritated in similar interpersonal situations. Moreover, because this primary anger has not been allowed completion of expression, the person is unaware of the adaptive action tendency and associated unmet needs and therefore does not act on her or his own behalf to get these needs met. Treatment, in such cases, involves focusing the anger on the specific significant other for the particular offenses. Expressing this anger to completion accesses the emotion scheme along with the unmet needs and maladaptive beliefs that generalize to other relationships. These beliefs can be examined and restructured in therapy and the person, more aware of those needs, can access internal and external resources for getting the needs met.

Client Example

A woman in therapy (discussed briefly early in this chapter) was diagnosed with major depressive disorder. Her symptoms included a fragile sense of self, such that she felt as if there was a "big empty space inside." She feared being without support and had a "bad temper" in which she would slam doors, break things, and fly into rages when her needs for understanding and support were not met. It was as if she interpreted lack of support as a sign of rejection or abandonment and that left her feeling alone, unloved, and unlovable, as well as desperate and helpless to change the situation. Lack of support was a threat to her self-integrity and will be discussed later (in Chapter 9) in terms of primary maladaptive anxiety. However, there also was an element of primary anger, particularly at her partner for unmet needs, for not attending to her, or taking her seriously. It was the intensity of her reaction that was inappropriate, and this partly seemed to be *generated* by unresolved issues and unexpressed anger toward her father.

Most of her early life, this client had been criticized, belittled, and dismissed by her father, who finally abandoned the family when she was a young teen. She had not seen or heard from him since. She had never been able to stand up for herself with him and continued to feel deeply angry for the way she had been treated. During one session, rather than explore the client's ongoing anger with her boyfriend for dismissing her, the therapist conjectured that being dismissed was intolerable and all too familiar to her. She suggested that they "put the anger where it belongs" and invited the client to imagine confronting her father in the empty chair. This was an opportunity to stand up for herself, to say all the things she had wanted to say as a child but couldn't. This was immensely empowering and left her feeling stronger and more confident in herself. Thus, focusing her anger *restructured* the maladaptive emotion scheme, which made her less vulnerable to being devastated by signs of lack of support in others and less chronically angry.

Secondary Anger at Unmet Dependency Needs and Interpersonal Threat

An example of secondary anger generated by interpersonal threat is seen in the aforementioned depressed client who chronically flew into a rage whenever she believed that she was not being heard or understood by her partner. The situation had been ongoing, she felt helpless to change it, and her anger was a reaction to this helplessness and frustration. It was important for the therapist first of all to acknowledge and validate her primary anger at not being heard as a kind of violation of her personhood. Also, part of the intervention strategy discussed above entailed redirecting her anger toward her abandoning father.

However, anger was her dominant response in most situations (her "temper" was one of the symptoms of her depression) and she seemed less in touch with other emotions. There was, as well, often a desperate and panicky quality to her expressions of anger, which suggested her underlying fear of dissolution and abandonment. This was consistent with discussions of her fragile sense of self and expressions of sadness and fear at unmet dependency needs.

After her reactive anger was acknowledged, an important repeated intervention involved refocusing on her underlying fear of abandonment (the generating condition for her secondary anger and bad feelings) and her sense of powerlessness. Having accessed the primary feeling, the underlying need and implicit belief were then identified and worked with.

The process of unpacking the secondary reaction and the cognitive–affective sequences associated with it involved exploring the fear generating her anger. This intervention strategy was described earlier in the section on process diagnosis of secondary anger. In therapy, as the client spoke angrily about feeling neglected by her partner, the therapist would redirect her attention to her primary fear by picking up her sense of feeling so uncared for. The therapist empathized with how desperate she felt, as though she couldn't survive without his support. Such a statement did not interpret her anger as a defensive reaction to fear, nor did it directly challenge the extremity of her anger reaction. Rather, it utilized empathy and the principle of present-centeredness to identify her current underlying feeling of fear and capture the intensity of her primary emotional experience. It refocused attention on her fear and the intensity of her need as the more core experience underlying her reactive anger. Going underneath the reactive anger to the more primary vulnerability is the key process in working with secondary anger.

CHAPTER EIGHT

Sadness and Distress

S ADNESS EMERGES FROM parting, separation, or loss of attachment. The psychological forms of separation include feeling left out or like we don't belong, being unable to communicate or express our true feelings, feeling neglected, and, of course, mourning the death or loss of a loved one. Sadness also can be evoked by disappointments or shattered hopes, failure to achieve important goals, and loss of self-esteem. Sadness can produce tears but differs from distress crying which is a general signal of suffering and a call for help. The distress is produced by other emotions, such as fear, shame, or anger. Crying acts as a signal that motivates the self and others to do something about the distressing circumstance. Distress is reduced by comfort in the form of soothing sounds, verbal reassurance, pacifiers, and physical contact.

Primary sadness needs to be distinguished from more complex experiences of pain, hurt, grief, and depression. Sadness is a discrete emotional state, compared to depression, which is a complex syndrome involving a variety of behaviors, thoughts, and feelings. Hurt is another complex feeling that lies in the domain of sadness but is not identical with it. Hurt is associated with rejection, feeling ignored, unrecognized, judged, and unvalued, and the tendency is either to withdraw or lash out. Pain, on the other hand, is the feeling of the self being damaged, wounded, or shattered. Finally, the complex process of grief involves sadness only when the loss is accepted as irrevocable and attempts to restore the loss, at least for the moment, are given up. The distress of sadness, at the core, is about the experience of irrevocable loss.

The two action tendencies associated with primary sadness are (1) reaching out to others for comfort and succor in order to reduce distress, and (2) withdrawal into self in order to recover from loss. Accordingly, sorrow inhibits the muscles and saps the energy. The head and eyes drop, facial muscles sag, and the voice becomes weak. A unique characteristic of the experience of sadness is its heaviness: people feel weighed down and move clumsily; holding themselves erect takes great effort; lying down and sometimes curling into a ball are preferred. Sadness involves "collapsing" into tears, passive withdrawal from involvement in life, momentary surrender, and letting go of the need for the lost object. There is nothing to be done but face the pain; struggling against and avoidance of pain simply prolongs suffering. Overall, tears of primary sadness are healing and bring with them a sense of exhaustion and relief. Sadness allows for acceptance of the loss, healing, and moving on to renewed interest in life. Acceptance of loss also enables the person to perceive the lost object more accurately or clearly, because perceptions are no longer clouded with the intensity of longing.

PROCESS DIAGNOSIS OF SADNESS AND DISTRESS

For the purpose of intervention, it is unnecessary to distinguish between the pain of sadness due to loss and other types of psychological pain. In all cases, the intervention strategy involves allowing and accepting the primary adaptive, although painful, emotion. However, it *is* clinically necessary to discriminate different types of crying, because distress crying can accompany a number of emotions in addition to primary sadness. Clients at the beginning of treatment are frequently highly distressed and cry easily and profusely about the things that are bothering them. However, they usually are not expressing primary sadness at loss but can be feeling angry, helpless, attempting to evoke support, or a combination of these. In these situations, interventions that simply promote allowing and accepting of the experience are not helpful. Thus, for the purpose of appropriate intervention, therapists need to distinguish between sadness and other emotional experiences, and between primary, secondary, and instrumental expressions of sadness.

Primary Adaptive Sadness

Primary adaptive sadness is a state that often appears in therapy as a brief moment embedded in a complex psychological process. It is characterized by a kind of momentary surrender or giving up and is free of blame. At other times it can be deeply and fully felt. In the early stages of therapy, primary adaptive sadness, like anger, is often either undifferentiated or suppressed. Obvious markers of suppressing sadness and emotional pain include intellectualization or minimizing damage and pain, tensing muscles, holding back tears, explicitly stated unwillingness to cry or go into the pain, along with fears or concerns about being overwhelmed by it.

Distinguishing primary sadness from secondary depression or victimized helplessness is based on knowledge of the situation and the person, as well as verbal and nonverbal cues including vocal quality, facial expression, and manner of experiencing. Above all, primary sadness, unlike helplessless and depression, is a lively state that leads to change. Recognizing undifferentiated sadness is done partly by knowledge of the triggering situation. For example, in situations of betrayal, sadness is mixed with anger; in situations of trauma, it is mixed with fear; sadness at abandonment can be mixed with fear and anger; sadness from abuse is mixed with anger, fear, and shame. All of these emotions can be primary, and each needs to be experienced and expressed completely. Interventions that differentiate sadness from these other emotions focus on the loss aspect of the situation.

Primary Maladaptive Sadness

The assessment of whether primary sadness is adaptive or maladaptive takes time and takes both the context and content of the sadness into account. If the situation involves loss and injury to self, the first step is to facilitate the experience and expression of the sadness in the belief that, over time, this will lead to a resolution of the emotion. In certain instances, however, the feeling doesn't seem to shift and the person repeats the same feeling again and again without any noticeable change in either quality or intensity. Alternatively, the sadness and tears can have a dysfunctional quality of fragmentation and fear, or helpless dependence with an inability to find a sense of internal coherence or agency. This suggests problems with underregulation of distress and a core sense of weakness. In these cases, the therapist and client begin to understand that this sadness is maladaptive and work toward restructuring this experience.

Pathological or complicated grief reactions can be examples of primary maladaptive sadness. The person is unable to cope with and move on from an important loss. Often, in these situations expression of unresolved anger and guilt and developing a stronger sense of self are found to be important. Some people feel inordinately sad at separations and avoid situations involving endings. Again, unresolved losses may be involved, and intervention entails accessing the emotion scheme and resolving the person's difficulties with accepting the loss. Finally, paradoxical sadness at gestures of kindness and tenderness from others, including the therapist, is a type of maladaptive primary sadness. It is as if kindness evokes deep longing, deprivation, and unmet dependency needs. Emotionally focused therapy (EFT) involves accessing the core emotion scheme or sense of self as one of feeling alone and unloved, acknowledging the pain and neediness, and then changing the scheme. This is accomplished partially through a corrective emotional experience with the therapist and partially through accessing alternate internal resources. The client needs to feel less deprived before she or he can tolerate kindness.

Secondary Sadness and Depression

It is important to distinguish between tears of primary sadness and pain, on the one hand, and tears that are in response to other emotional experiences, such as frustration, hopelessness, or anger. This occurs when clients chronically collapse into hurt, victimization, and sadness whenever they feel angry. Secondary reactions are recognizable by verbal cues and their temporal sequence—for example, when anger first is expressed, followed by tears. Exploration of these experiences in therapy reveals that the tears are precipitated by secondary cognitive–affective processes such as anticipation of loss or rejection that results in fear, distress, and sad feelings.

The most common secondary reaction associated with sadness is depression, which involves a kind of generalized hopelessness rather than genuine acceptance of loss. Thus, depressed people will express resignation about loss or injury to self, such as "What is the point in crying over spilled milk?" Self-critical and "should" statements also can result in people feeling defeated, hopeless, and sad. In these cases, the sadness is secondary to a complex cognitive–affective sequence. When lingering depression results from stifled primary sadness at loss, or any other primary experience, treatment involves unpacking the secondary depressive reaction into its underlying cognitive–affective determinants, and acknowledging and experiencing the painful primary emotion. Interventions help the client sink into the hopeless bad feelings in order to access alternate internal resources so that the feelings shift. The client then is able to acknowledge and accept a specific loss and move on to new concerns.

Instrumental Sadness

More instrumental expressions of sadness are observed when people cry because they are feeling helpless or dependent, or as an aspect of complaining. This is pejoratively referred to as "whining" and is the case when tears are a form of protest, expressing how poorly treated the person feels, with the hope that it will evoke sympathy, support, or understanding. People may or may not be aware of the instrumental function of their tears and can be genuinely needy. However, this sadness does not primarily result from an experience of loss and often does not elicit the desired support. Instrumental tears that function to get attention from others, to avoid self-care, or as an excuse to stop functioning need to be modified. It is appropriate to empathically challenge or interpret the function of instrumental tears in order to access the underlying motivations and needs, and teach the client better ways to get her or his needs met.

EMOTIONALLY FOCUSED INTERVENTION

Solutions to the problems of pain and sadness come by allowing and accepting the pain, and experiencing and expressing it, in order to live through it and come out the other end. However, people must have confidence in their ability to carry on and that things will get better, if they are to allow themselves to accept a major loss. Our approach provides the support necessary to complete this work of grieving, to allow the person to surrender, withdraw, and recuperate, and to help the person learn to comfort him- or herself. EFT interventions also access longing for contact and comfort from others and promote seeking that contact outside of therapy.

Loss of attachment is extremely painful, and for some people inability to regulate the self and remain intact after loss results in problems. Such losses can include acute and situational loneliness, adjustment to death or divorce, alienation associated with depressive states, and the chronic loneliness and alienation of people with long-standing interpersonal difficulties. Social skills training and group therapy for those with skills deficits can help people make needed connections with others, and distress tolerance skills can help clients cope with painfully lonely circumstances. However, it also is critically important to acknowledge the sadness and pain of loneliness and separation in order to mobilize the desire and action tendency toward connection.

Our approach includes changing maladaptive cognitions that fuel depression. However, we do not directly challenge cognitions because these are viewed as by-products of more complex emotion schemes and core experiences. Rather, change is accomplished by accessing and fully experiencing feelings of hopelessness, and/or unpacking the cognitive–affective components of depression in order to access underlying primary adaptive experience and healthy re-sources—in this case, those related to sadness. These then act to restructure core maladaptive self-related emotion schemes and challenge maladaptive cognitions.

Intervention Principles Relevant to Sadness

As we stated in Chapter 7, all of the EFT intervention principles are used in therapeutic work with all of the emotions, but the following principles are especially important in working with sadness.

Direct Attention to Internal Experience (Bodily Felt Sense)

Sadness is an inwardly moving experience characterized by passivity or inaction. Thus empathic responses that capture and highlight this quiet quality are relied on more than active interventions. The therapist is usually less active in order to allow the client to withdraw. However, sadness is certainly accessed in the context of enactments such as chair work and imagery. When, for a fleeting moment, clients' eyes well up with tears, the therapist can respond with "Something about that touches you; can you stay with that feeling?" When clients speak about situations of loss or hurt, questions about where it hurts and empathic responses that reflect the feeling of ache, pain, or brokenness, the "big empty space" or hole inside, lifelessness, or a desire to give in, surrender, collapse, or stay in bed can direct attention to bodily experiences of primary sadness.

Interventions, then, help clients symbolize the meaning of the experience—what the pain or emptiness, the lump in the throat, heaviness in the chest are about. Clients are encouraged to "speak from" their tears, say what is missing or was missed, what weighs them down, and how this loss affected or affects them in their current lives.

Present-Centeredness

Tracking moment-by-moment experience is critical when one is working with sadness because the experience of primary sadness can be so fleeting. As we noted in Chapter 7, clients can move quickly from sadness to anger, to fear, and denial, and back to sadness, in working through an important loss. Therapists do not want to force a premature closure or acceptance of loss, and even a moment of deep weeping can be followed by mobilization of anger or numbness. In the midst of anger expression, the client may become suddenly quiet and withdrawn, and the therapist needs to ask what is going on for him or her at that moment: "What's happening on the inside?"

An important part of the present-centeredness principle concerns empathic affirmation of a client's sense of vulnerability, of feeling weak and exposed when experiencing pain and sadness. Responses at these moments, such as "Yes, this is where it hurts," or "It hurts a lot," or "It's very sad to think about those times," or "Feeling so utterly alone," are not intended to explore, deepen, or intensify experience but to validate it, to metaphorically hold the client and allow him or her to sink into the warded-off sadness. This art of being with someone who is grieving, comforting them with your presence without trying to fix or solve the problem or make the pain go away, can be difficult for novice therapists. In working with sadness and pain, therapists need to develop the capacity to allow themselves to be deeply touched by the suffering of others and not move away from the pain.

Intensifying Experience

Intensification is designed to overcome avoidance of sadness, to heighten awareness to the point where it's difficult to deny, so the person lets go of control, feels the pain, and grieves over the loss. Sadness can be deepened through the use of metaphors, connotative language, and evocative empathic reflections. People can weep silently or deeply. Responses that direct attention to poignancy, bodily experiences of aching or emptiness, metaphors of brokenness, cutting, or longing, and references to children and childhood can be powerfully evocative. For example, paradoxical sadness or pain that occurs in response to kindness, nurturing, or caring on the part of therapist can be deepened with responses such as "Somehow it touches a deep longing (or emptiness) inside," or "So much pain, so many unmet needs," or "Feeling like a needy little child, starved for love." Also, enactments of nurturing, soothing, comforting the "little child" part of the self, or actually stroking a pillow or other transitional object can be powerfully evocative and deepen the experience of sadness. The popular "inner child" movement has incorporated use of transitional soothing objects such as teddy bears to symbolize the small, sad child and heighten awareness of unresolved hurt, loss, and unmet attachment needs. Likewise, expressing longing for love, physical affection, and comfort from an imagined loved one can deepen the sadness experience. Sobbing and weeping also can be facilitated by massaging neck and shoulder muscles to release muscular tension.

THERAPEUTIC EPISODES WORKING
WITH SADNESS AND PAIN

The same situations that evoke anger also can evoke sadness; thus, the following episodes on sadness involve clients presented in the previous chapter. It appeared that, for some of these clients, experience and full expression of previously constricted primary anger associated with the troubling situation enabled them to let go of blame and move into acknowledgement and expression of their hurt and sadness. If one views sadness in terms of grieving, these clients were able to complete the earlier protest stage in the grieving process and move into a later acceptance stage. They felt empowered and better able to accept the loss. However, the reverse sequence also is possible, where expression of sadness then leads to the acknowledgement of previously constricted anger.

The following subsections describe several types of sadness experience that illustrate different EFT intervention strategies: (1) sadness at interpersonal loss and deprivation; (2) sadness at loss of identity; (3) complicated grief associated with death; (4) pain, distress, and sadness from trauma or abuse; and (5) secondary sadness and depression. Again, the eight steps of the EFT process (Chapter 6) and the intervention principles will be included in the clinical examples.

Sadness at Deprivation or Loss

In its broadest sense, the interruption or overcontrol of sadness results in an inability to complete the work of grieving. People will not allow themselves to cry and instead firm themselves up by constricting their breathing and tightening chest, throat, and facial muscles. Sadness sometimes is interrupted because people are busy dealing with other survival problems or do not have the necessary safe place or support to let down their guard, be vulnerable, and give themselves over to healing. In these cases, it often is easier to be angry because anger is empowering, helps to shore them up, and enables them to carry on. Anger also plays a role in the overcontrol of sadness in power-struggle situations. People often refuse to acknowledge or show the other how weak or hurt they are because of internalized injunctions against weakness or lack of trust.

Others control sadness because of a learned Pollyanna view (e.g., that it's "a comfort to look on the bright side") or because of a fatalistic attitude (e.g., that it's "God's will" that one suffer). Others have injunctions against "wallowing in self-pity." There are many cultural injunctions against displays of sadness or grief. People are encouraged to be brave or stoic, keep a "stiff upper lip," not be a "crybaby" or a sissy, or "grin and bear it." Such cultural and family injunctions can contribute to a general fear of and inability to acknowledge emotional vulnerability and sadness at loss.

In situations of loss both primary anger and sadness are associated with injuries to self-esteem and unresolved disappointments in relationships with parents or in adult attachment relationships. One of the goals of therapy is to differentiate the anger and sadness in these situations and have each fully experienced, expressed, and worked through. It is important for therapists to recognize that in these situations both sadness and anger can be primary and need to be validated and deepened in therapy in order to access the adaptive components of each.

The present-centeredness principle, as a guideline in working with loss, states that the experience that is most alive should be given priority and focused on. However, clients need more help with accessing the emotion that is more difficult for them to acknowledge and express. Accessing the most deeply and frequently inhibited primary emotional experience enhances growth for the person and makes accessible new and adaptive information. Thus, in the therapeutic episodes that follow, the process diagnosis was that unacknowledged or suppressed primary sadness and distress was the client's most salient experience at the moment, and that full experiential acknowledgement of the primary sadness would be most beneficial and growth enhancing for the client.

The masking of sadness by both primary and secondary anger and the importance of focusing on the least available emotion was vividly illustrated in therapy with a 7-year-old boy. This child had been abandoned by his mother and been shuffled from foster home to foster home. He had been abandoned, rejected, betrayed, and deprived of love all his life and had told his therapist that "no one loves me." He had temper tantrums every time his current foster parents said "no" to him, and part of his therapy involved emotion awareness training. In one of the exercises he was asked what a person is feeling when he or she says, "I hate you," something he says to his foster parents during his tantrums. This child responded that the person is feeling "sad." Undoubtedly, this child experiences both anger and sadness about being abandoned, but he predominantly expresses anger; even his sadness is expressed as secondary anger. If he grows up to be a man who is unable to acknowledge his primary pain and sadness and has no skills for accurately symbolizing and communicating his emotional experience, his needs for love and connection will never be met. His anger will push others away rather than "pull for" the nurturance and succorance he desires.

The following case example illustrates work with primary sadness when both anger and sadness are present.

Client Example

A client who had been abandoned by her husband some 20 years earlier wanted companionship and the intimacy of a relationship "before I get much older" but found herself pushing away potential partners. She was fearful of allowing anyone to get close enough to hurt her and shatter her life as it had been when her husband walked out on her and their four small children. She described herself as being in a state of shock at the time, and struggling to keep her head above water and keep life going for herself and her children. She had coped by shoring herself up, controlling her emotions, and not allowing herself to feel the pain because she feared falling apart. She did not have a safe time and place to let down her guard. This was reinforced by well-intentioned friends who cautioned, "Don't shed one tear over that bastard. He's not worth it." She had limited support and was responding to the demands of her situation. She had never expressed her intense anger at her ex-husband for the pain and hardship he had caused not only in leaving but for what she perceived as his lack of caring and his self-centeredness throughout their marriage. Therapy provided a safe place for her to express these things and for grieving that had been postponed for 20 years, as well as to help her restructure her fears about getting involved again in an intimate relationship.

In the following therapy excerpt, expression of anger at her ex-husband spontaneously and quickly shifted to accessing her pain and to deep weeping for the devastation and intense vulnerability she felt at the time he left. Interventions included acknowledging and validating her pain by empathically affirming her vulnerability with responses such as "It feels almost unbearable," rather than attempting to explore or intensify her experience at this point. This also is an example of how sadness that is devastating often is mixed with fear of not being able to cope with the pain. In the session, the client has been describing her husband's behavior during their marriage:

ACCESS PRIMARY ANGER

T: So you resent his selfishness. [Promote ownership and agency]

C: I not only resent it, but I hate him for it, I really do! I hate him for that! ... The word isn't strong enough even to say how much I hate him.

T: Try saying it louder, and imagine saying it to him, "I hate you!" [Intensify]

C: I *hate* you. How can anybody hate anybody so much? I didn't think I had that much hate in me (*clenches fists*).

T: What would you like to do with those clenched fists? It seems important to express that as fully as you can, such a strong feeling. [Analyze expression]

C: I feel like I'd like to pound something, yeah.

T: Here, (*brings chair and pillow closer to client*) try pounding, go ahead ... really make that fist. That seems like a powerful feeling you have, let's express it (*models pounding chair*). [Intensify]

C: I don't know ... I don't really even know how to do that. I don't know that.

T: That's OK, just start—I hate your selfishness, I hate what you did to me—whatever words fit (*models pounding*).

C: (*starts vigorously pounding pillow on chair*)

T: Yeah, good, yes, yes, what would you like to say? Put some words to this, how dare you, I'd like to kill you, you bastard, anything ... (C: *Stops pounding.*) What's happening? [Focus on present]

ACCESS AND SUPPORT EXPRESSION OF PRIMARY SADNESS

C: (*pause*) I've just got such a strong emotion in me, I can't ...

T: Yeah, it's OK, stay with your feeling, (C: *Begins crying.*) yeah, let it come. Yeah, yeah, let it come (C: *Deeply sobbing*. T: *Begins massaging client's shoulders.*) Yes, such a lot of pain, years and years of it ... mm-humm ... it's OK, let it come.... (C: *Sobbing.*) ... It hurts ... mm-humm ... all those losses, all those years ... mm-humm, mm-humm

C: (*sobbing*) How can anybody hurt anybody so much? How can they? And then walk away without even feeling any emotion out of it.

T: Such a ... just hurts absolutely to the quick ... mm-humm, mm-humm, (C: *Sobs.*) mm-humm, right to the depths of your soul

... (C: *Stops crying.*) Can you tell me what's happening for you? [Focus on present-centeredness, Direct attention]

ARTICULATE MALADAPTIVE BELIEFS

C: ... I'm trying to figure out how somebody can do what he did and just walk away and not feel anything. Does he not have a conscience? ... He is just nothing in my eyes, just nothing, and I guess it bothers me how I allowed it to happen—how did I allow it to happen? Why would anyone keep coming back for more.

T: That seems important, too. Let's spend some time trying to understand how you could have been so vulnerable.... How are you feeling right now? [Direct attention, Establish intentions]

C: Well, I'm feeling very tired, but I feel some relief, I feel like I've got something, like I feel like I got something out of here (*hand on gut*), I feel, um, I just feel kinda relieved.

Thus, accessing and expressing her deep anger and sadness also accessed maladaptive self-blame and beliefs that somehow she "allowed" this to happen. These beliefs were contributing to her fear of intimacy and were now available for exploration and *restructuring*. Later in therapy, the client and the therapist were able to draw on her current resources to challenge and restructure the fear that she would repeat this desperation and lack of assertion in another relationship. This process will be presented in Chapter 9 on fear and distress.

Client Example

The following example illustrates work with avoidance of the sadness and pain of many adult losses and feeling unloved as a child. This avoidance of pain was assessed as one of the *underlying determinants* of client "L.'s" depression and alienation. Early in treatment she had been surprised by the therapist's use of the word "pain" to symbolize her experience; she had never thought of her experience that way. She found it difficult to experience her pain and how truly victimized she had been, at times, in her life. She had been socially anxious and felt isolated all her life, and had been in a number of unhappy and abusive adult relationships. She was painfully lonely—"Sometimes I'm climbing the walls, I'm so lonely"—needed contact and comfort, needed to communicate her desire for companionship, and to overcome her fear of doing so. Heightening her awareness of sadness and acknowledging pain were the means of achieving these objectives.

There were frequent markers of feeling embarrassed about being hurt and sad, such as "I don't want to be teary" or "It's embarrassing to be hurt." Additionally, she expressed paradoxical sadness when her eyes welled up with tears in response to the therapist's empathic, caring responses. The therapist reflected that "something touched you just now," and the client responded, in a "little girl" tone of voice, while sitting on her hands, that she could not "tolerate kindness from others." Subsequent interventions helped her attend to and symbolize that experience: "intolerable . . . like it hurts"; "like it touches a sore spot inside"; "kindness is somehow painful . . . you end up feeling like a desperately needy little girl?" The last response illustrates how analyzing the expressive quality in the client's tone of voice and bodily posture led to increased awareness and experience. When the therapist asked about her memories of kindness as a child, there were none; she recalled only deprivation, lack of love, and invalidation. The therapist again directed attention to her unmet primary need by responding that as a child, she must have longed for some kindness and how painful it must have been not to get it.

This triggered episodic memories of events with her mother. She was particularly distressed by what she perceived to be her mother's indifference to her suffering as a child. For example, her mother watched while her father beat her, asked her to leave the country when she became pregnant as a teenager, and constantly invalidated her experience. She realized how she came to believe that her own feelings and perceptions were not to be trusted and that there must be something wrong with her. This left her unable to communicate, isolated, cut off, and painfully alone. Deep pain and sadness, which she had been unable to express, was under her fear and confusion.

The following excerpt, from Session 4, illustrates exploration of her overcontrol of experience and working with her sadness. The client has been speaking about a time her parents were visiting:

ACCESS SADNESS AND NEED

C: I was alone at the time, with the children, and I wanted them to stay with me, but they stayed with my brother.

T: So they were there and you wanted, or needed, some kind of help. [Establish need]

C: Just a bit of comfort, just that they thought of me or something, I think, would have been good enough.

T: Yeah, some acknowledgment or comfort, that must have been very hurtful for you.

C: It was as if she was unable to see the need or do anything about it, or didn't want to see it, or didn't have the sensitivity to see it. It seems that she really didn't have an awful lot of interest in me.

T: So you felt like she didn't really care about you. . . . What were some of the things you would have liked? It seems important to put those things in words, what you missed. [Symbolize]

C: I don't know what I missed, anything would have done, (*weeps . . .*) anything at all would have done.

T: Yeah, stay with that—I really needed her to care. [Establish need]

C: That was the second time that happened; first time was when I was pregnant and I wasn't married and I didn't know what to do. . . . When I phoned and told her, she said I wasn't to dare to come into the country.

T: You must have felt so rejected. What would you have liked her to do, as your mother? [Establish need]

C: She could have at least not stood in my way, some kind of human care and attention. This sounds so . . . I don't know. (*sits up in her seat and frowns evaluatively*)

ACCESS INTERRUPTIVE COGNITIONS

T: What happens as you say that? Something stopped you. [Focus on present]

C: I'm thinking to myself, it sounds so juvenile, and so self-pitying and stuff like that; it sounds like I'm whining.

T: That sounds like another part of you, shutting you down, passing judgment on your feelings. Can you get in touch with that part of yourself: "Stop feeling sorry for yourself"? Something happened there that stopped you from feeling sad. [Direct attention]

C: Yeah, I heard my own voice.

T: So that's what happened. So do what you just did if you can. How did you stop yourself from feeling those feelings, like your own voice said stop being so childish? What else did you say?

C: You sound whiny, miserable, yuk, gross, sniveling, especially with things that are past and dead.

T: So what should she do, L., "come off it"?

C: Forget it, stop thinking about it, stop looking for pity or sympathy. I was thinking the other day that nobody gives a damn—you can't expect people to be even remotely interested in my situation or circumstance.

ACCESS INTERNAL RESOURCES TO CHALLENGE INTERRUPTIONS

T: So its this sense that no one cares or is interested, so what should L. do with her sadness, just?

C: (*pause*) Suffer in silence, 'cause there's no point. But I have to get it out.

T: Uh-huh, I have to get it out.

C: How do I get rid of this voice? Somehow I must get rid of this, I'll die if I don't. (*weeps*) I want to live, I want peace, something nice.

T: Yeah, some peace, some comfort, free of this burden, it seems like you have a lot of tears to cry, a lot of pain to work through ... like you never got the mothering you needed. [Symbolize, Establish need]

C: How do I fill the void? How do you ever get over that? (*weeps*)

The therapist responds that this is a basic human need that won't go away, and stresses the importance of the client finding other ways to fill the need and of working on it, in this individual therapy and possibly in group therapy. The client remarks that she has always liked older women and thinks that perhaps they represent the mother she never had. The therapist supports her search for nurturing women in her life and validates that she can grow, as an adult, from those kinds of adult connections.

The following transcript is from a later session in which the therapist helps the client overcome interruption of her sadness by supporting the emergence of primary needs. Again, she has been talking about her relationship with her mother.

ACKNOWLEDGE AND VALIDATE EXPERIENCE

C: (*sigh*) ... I mean the words in my mind are that I don't like talking about it. But I don't know whether that's true or not, you know.

T: So it's hard to talk about it, especially to talk . . .

C: I don't know *who* I would talk to, I mean, I wouldn't talk to anybody at all, except you. I might say, I don't get along with my mother, or my mother and I are not close, but I wouldn't go into it.

EVOKE/AROUSE BAD FEELINGS

T: In an ideal world, and if you could say what was in your heart to your mother. What would you say? [Symbolize]

C: Oh, nothing. I would just say, you never speak to me.

T: The pain is so great I need to push you away.

C: Never, ever, ever speak to me.

T: It hurts so much.

C: I couldn't utter those words. *Never!* (*sniffles*)

T: You couldn't tell her about your pain. (C: *Sniffles.*) . . . Like you wanted so much from her that you never could get [Establish need]

C: *No!* I wouldn't want to utter those words. Never. (*sniffles*) She just put me right outside the human race for all my life (*blows nose*). . . . (*pause*) . . . this is ridiculous.

T: What's happening? You feel . . . how could I be so hurt still? [Focus on present]

C: I don't know. Now why would I say it's ridiculous, because it's not ridiculous, is it?

T: No. No, it's not ridiculous. This is who you are at this moment.

C: There's nothing I can do about it. . . . Really and truly, I mean even writing a letter to her is more than I would want to do. (T: Hmm.) I guess it seems, it's funny, it seems worse as far as my mother is concerned and less so, as far as my father's concerned, and it was him I feared all my life (*blows nose*). . . .

ACCESS THE CORE MALADAPTIVE EMOTION SCHEME, PRIMARY SADNESS, AND NEEDS

C: I just felt so terrified, so unprotected. I remember trying to disappear, to not be seen. I would just slink away like a dog when he came in the room—I felt so alone, I needed protection, I needed a mother, I felt so alone.

T: So sort of like you desperately needed her and the fact that she wasn't there has just cut you to the quick. (C: *Sniffles.*) It's unbearable almost—desperately needed a mother. [Establish needs]

C: It would seem so unfair to put all the burden on her . . . but I can't do otherwise.

T: Can't do otherwise for some reason. (C: *Sniffles.*) She's who you needed. She is . . .

C: I could have dealt with the rest. . . . I'm sure I could have dealt with the rest, I mean there was nothing nice about it, but it would have been bearable. It was even bearable. I guess it must've been bearable, I bore it.

T: So if she'd been there for me, I would've, it would've made all the difference in the world. [Refocus attention]

C: It would have been . . . I mean, I *imagine* anyway. I would *imagine* (*blows nose*).

T: Sounds like you needed that more than anything. (C: *Blows nose again.*) [Establish needs]

C: If that, if that had been available to me, somehow or another, support, I might have floated off the planet, it would have been so much more . . . humane. Something like that. (T: Hmm.) . . . I don't know.

T: It makes sense what you're saying. It makes perfect, perfect sense.

C: And yet I understand from my own experience that you do all you can. I mean I have seen my children go without. And it has torn me. And yet I've been unable to do anything for them.

FACILITATE RESTRUCTURING

T: Sounds like you're . . . sounds like you had a sudden glimpse of what it was like for her—I tried, I did what I could but I just . . . What would she say, I wonder?

C: I guess she might say she too felt trapped and was doing the best she could. But I needed support and she didn't give it to me. I don't forgive her . . . but I feel sad . . . sad about what I never had. I have to get on with it though. Fifty years of suffering is enough—I want to get on with what I have left of my years.

This primary emotional experience helped mobilize her deep longing for connection with others and helped her to articulate how her fear and confusion had interfered with her awareness and ability to express this part of herself. This accessing of her sadness and of the action tendency to connect also motivated her to persist in therapy, to face her painful memories, and to seek out, with the therapist's help, an ongoing social skills therapy group. She was determined to change her life. Throughout, the therapist validated her strengths at surviving, despite her suffering, and supported her capacity for self-care. The therapist helped her draw on her experience as a parent to identify her own unmet childhood needs and feel confident about their validity. She needed a lot of guidance and support, balanced with more active exploration. The therapeutic relationship was an important source of new interpersonal learning that she could trust someone and receive understanding and comfort.

Sadness at Loss of Identity

In situations involving losses of self-identity or esteem, people frequently minimize the importance of the loss and underestimate the severity and the difficulty in healing. This attitude is reinforced in cultures that tend to value stoicism and strength. For example, people are reluctant to "feel sorry" for themselves and minimize the losses associated with health problems, changes in lifestyle, choosing to have an abortion, or leave a relationship. One crucial aspect of EFT is validation of the significance of client injuries and losses and the associated pain and sadness, thus giving the person "permission" to grieve. Symbolizing the meaning of the loss aids in the creation of new meaning and self-identity. The following case example illustrates this type of therapeutic work.

A woman sought therapy because of difficulty adjusting to her limitations following a heart attack. This was 2 years following the crisis, and her condition was physically controlled but she was chronically depressed. It was established in therapy that ungrieved losses of her career and way of life—her identity as a strong, competent, independent woman—were among the underlying determinants of her depression. She minimized her situation with beliefs such as "Im lucky compared to some others" and attitudes developed by a lifetime of being strong and seeing weakness as "self-indulgent wallowing." This view of herself as wallowing also was exacerbating her depression. Therapy was complicated by her inability to tolerate stress due to fragile health. Thus she feared the stress of reexperiencing the pain of her heart attack if she connected with her loss, and the stress of reopening old wounds and parental injuries that were triggered by her current vulnerability.

Therapy needed to be safe; the client set the pace while *exploring* her bad feelings and acknowledging the death of part of herself, giving it importance and dignity rather than minimizing it. The therapist encouraged her to symbolize specific losses, saying, "You survived but a big part of you died, by the sounds of it." Talking about all the things she missed, such as loss of her creative self, her active, strong, and independent self, *accessed* her emotional pain. She had always coped by distracting herself with hard work, but now even her usual coping strategy was unavailable to her. Through therapist empathic affirmation and validation of her experience, she was able to acknowledge these losses and weep for herself. The therapist helped her create rituals to say goodbye to her old life and to make way for something new and, at the same time, validated that there would be times when she would feel the pain of loss, she would be excruciatingly aware of being a "one-legged woman," and would need to cry. The client accepted that her loss would never completely go away but that she could rebuild her life. *Restructuring* or *creation of new meaning* by redefining herself, rather than clinging to the past, was only possible by facing the void that these losses had created and clarifying the significance of what had been lost.

Resolving Complicated Grief

Sometimes clients have been unable to complete grieving for the death or loss of a loved one, because the relationship was complicated by unresolved feelings of guilt, anger, or pain. For example, the client in Chapter 7 whose mother committed suicide was unable to forgive her mother and see her death as anything other than rejection and abandonment. Similarly, clients find it difficult to grieve for the death of an abusive parent when the relationship was complicated by the pain of unmet attachment needs and anger at abuse. Another client was riddled with guilt about being abusive toward her elderly mother; she was unable to forgive herself, fully grieve over the loss, and move on. These clinical examples illustrate the connection between sadness, shame, guilt, and anger in pathological grief reactions. Emotionally focused grief work involves differentiating, acknowledging, and expressing all these facets of the experience. Empty-chair work can be beneficial in enabling the client to say what she or he was unable to say in the relationship and to say good-bye.

In helping clients work through the loss of a loved one, the therapist needs to help mourners review their relationship with the dead person, going over and over scenes of disappointment and disagreement, and touching lightly on those of joy and pride. As in the previous example, the therapist acknowledges the irrevocability of the loss and the difficulty of acceptance, despite healing and building a new life, and simultaneously helps the client to create new meaning of how the lost relationship fits into his or her present life. This is done by symbolizing what is missed, what the needs are that must be met in some other way.

Client Example

A client's mother died of cancer when she was a teenager. Grieving for her mother was incomplete and complicated by what the client referred to as "covert sexual abuse" by her father. She had been her father's confidante and ally against her mother, and together she and her father had rejected her mother. As a teenager, she believed that she did not love her mother and her mother did not love her. She even refused to attend her mother's funeral, claiming that she would not be a hypocrite. It was when she had her own child that she changed. She recalled holding her infant son and being overwhelmed with love for him and suddenly realizing that her mother must have felt the same toward her. She had been unable to come to terms with her guilt, to grieve for her mother's death and the lost opportunity for a relationship with her.

In therapy, in the process of working through the issues of anger and dependency with her father, she experienced and expressed the grief, regret, and love toward her mother that she had previously disallowed. Expressing her sorrow and believing that her mother would forgive her alleviated her guilt and allowed her to forgive herself and emotionally restructure her relationship with her mother. An important intervention was evocation of memories of herself when her mother was sick and dying. This helped her reexperience her own feelings toward her mother, imagine how painful it must have been for the mother to be rejected by her, and access her feelings of neediness for her father's attention and approval.

The following transcript is from Session 7 and illustrates the resolution of complicated grief by symbolizing new meaning. The client began the session by recounting a dream in which she was caring for her sick mother.

ACKNOWLEDGE AND EXPLORE BAD FEELINGS

C: I know it will always be a point of sadness because I wasn't the way I would have liked to have been during it, so I'm kind of living it vicariously now, which is not the same thing as doing the right thing at the right time.

T: So there's a sense of missed opportunity—it was there and somehow you weren't in the right place to be able to take advantage of that. (C: Yeah.) So its like, in the dream, you're sort of giving yourself another chance. [Symbolize]

C: Yeah, and that's how I really felt it. . . . It was kind of a vindication of not having done it before, knowing that I could have done it if things hadn't been the way they were. I think it was a sort of forgiveness, that it wasn't my fault. . . . She understood, and it was me being hard on myself about it.

T: So you've been feeling quite guilty or responsible for not having given her some care and love. [Promote agency and ownership]

C: Or any level of compassion or sympathy, just a real lot of disdain and hatred during that period, that she should get it over with, and die, so the rest of us could get on with our lives . . . and being able to have my dad to myself. . . .

Access Emotion Meaning

T: I feel that the way for us to go is to reevoke that time around when your mom died. I wonder what would happen if you went back to when you were 16 and, in imagination, interact with her as you saw her then. In a way we'll reevoke the situation, but we're gonna take it further and give you a chance to see what is left from then that is unfinished. . . . We can't change the reality, but we can change, somewhat, how things sit with us. [Evoke memory, Provide rationale]

C: . . . I realize my mom really *did* do a lot of things out of love and I just wasn't able to appreciate it because of this other overbearing person who in some sense wouldn't let me be close to her.

T: Maybe start by putting your father in the chair and tell him—it sounds like what you're saying is "Let me have my mom" or "Get out of my way" or something. Can you remember back to that period and picture him and you, as you were, and, as yourself, as that young girl, tell him . . . [Focus on present]

(*Client talks about conflicting feelings toward mother and father and wanting her father's attention but now resenting his interfering with her relationship with her mother.*)

ACCESS PRIMARY SADNESS AND NEED

T: So what you couldn't say to him then was ... I needed you but I also needed my mom, I needed her love. [Establish need]

C: I needed her (*sobs*), I still need her (*sobs deeply*).

T: Of course you do. Why don't you put her here and tell her that?

C: Mom, I need you, I love you, and this is all I can do now 'cause I can't change what was, (*sniffle*) and I feel like it's not really enough, but it's all I can do, and it wasn't my fault.

T: Does it make sense to tell her I miss you? [Symbolize]

C: Yeah, I do miss you.

T: Tell her some of the things you miss. [Symbolize]

C: I wish you were around to help me with G. [son], 'cause sometimes it really gets too much, it's too hard. It would be nice to have your help, someone who I could trust and know would really love him and take care of him, or give me advice. . . . I feel like she didn't want to leave us.

T: Come over here and be your mom and tell A. [the client] about leaving. [Focus on present]

C: (*switches chairs, enacts mother*) I didn't want to leave you, and I was really afraid that your dad wouldn't be able to look after you. . . . I loved you (*sobs*). . . . I was so sad that you couldn't love me back (*blows nose*).

RESTRUCTURING

T: I wonder what else you can say to help A. understand, or what it was like for you. [Symbolize]

C: I feel like I knew what your father was doing to you, but I was powerless to do anything. You were so, you thought you were so close to him, and you were just doing what you wanted, and you were so strong in doing that, and I knew that I couldn't do anything or say anything to change what was (*turns to therapist*). And I think that was probably really true.

T: So I couldn't be strong for you. [Refocus]

C: Yeah, I was really powerless, I couldn't be more than I was, 'cause I had my own stuff, I felt dominated by him too. I was very unused to asserting myself 'cause that wasn't in my history. I just wanted to do things that would make him love me, and really I was behaving like a child too. . . .

(Therapist directs client to switch to "self" chair and respond to imagined mother.)

C: I can see that you felt like a little girl and that the sicker you became the more helpless you became and more childlike, looking to him to take care of you. . . .

T: How did you feel seeing her like that? [Direct attention]

C: I guess I felt kind of angry. (T: Tell her.) I wanted you to be a grown up and not a child. . . . I wish you and dad had dealt with your own stuff. . . . I understand that you already had a big history of subordination and (*sobs*) being expected to be the good little girl.

T: What are your tears about? [Focus on present, Symbolize]

C: Well, I just know how hard that is to combat.

T: So sometimes I just want to give up and be helpless too? [Promote ownership and agency]

C: Well, I do, and that's why sometimes I want to just give up on G. [son] (*weeps*), just a heavy burden. . . . It made me grow up too fast. . . .

T: There's still a lot of feeling there—what's it like for you to make contact with your parents like this? [Direct attention, Symbolize]

C: I dunno, it's just such a lost opportunity that we can't replace. Sometimes I think she felt lonely and disconnected in the relationship, and felt my father's animosity, and grew her own animosity toward him, and felt disillusioned with her life and her children, and all the things that were supposed to have meaning.

T: Is there something that you'd like to say to her about that, like you wish. . . ? [Establish need]

C: Well, I wanna say, (*to empty chair*) I wish I'd been able to give you the love that you needed too, but I couldn't. . . . The situation must have just looked hopeless to you. I don't blame her for dying—she just didn't see any other way out. I know how I feel when G. [son] is mean to me.

Support Self-Affirming Stance

T: I think the tragedy is that if only she had lived longer you could have given each other that support and love.

C: Yeah, I think that's true. . . . I don't know if I've had a chance to really face the loss and the grief before.

Thus restructuring and the *creation of new meaning* came about by fully acknowledging the mutual sadness and tragedy of their loss, expressing regret at her part in the situation, and coming to believe that her mother could understand her needs and, although she was very sad, she would forgive her.

Grieving Losses Associated with Trauma or Abuse

Treating the effects of trauma and abuse involves helping clients not only express their anger but grieve for their irrevocable losses, the damage to self. Again, one of the hallmarks of trauma is shattering of fundamental and valued assumptions around which one has constructed a meaningful life and identity.

With trauma, the fundamental sense of self-coherence and assumptions about reality are shattered or broken, and the self is deeply wounded. This often leads to a natural avoidance of pain. Avoidance of psychological pain becomes a problem, however, when the avoidance becomes chronic, interferes with the healing process, and prolongs suffering. This is often the case with some forms of pathological grief and posttraumatic stress disorder in which the inability to acknowledge painful losses or psychic injuries perpetuate the symptoms. The avoidance of the pain keeps people stuck, unable to create new meaning and integrate new information, so that the maladaptive emotion scheme related to the traumatic loss cannot evolve. Psychic wounds cannot heal, and the person is vulnerable to these wounds being continually reopened. Thus, the person becomes guarded, self-protective, vigilant, fragile, and isolated. Fear of the pain comes to rule his or her life and relationships. It is this that must be overcome in treatment.

In working with clients who have been emotionally, physically, or sexually abused, pain and sadness often emerge when clients are talking about the scars, the effects, and the consequences of the abuse on their lives, rather than when talking about the situation itself. The latter is accompanied more by feelings of anger, fear, disgust, and shame. It is only after the fact that one becomes aware of what has been lost, the hurtful impact, including the loss of innocence, security, love and protection, and the loss of close relationships with other family members because trust was shattered and sexuality was damaged. Interventions intended to help clients access and express primary sadness need to specifically focus on connecting with such experiences of injury and loss, rather than on reexperiencing details of the abusive situation itself. Often these losses are minimized or the loss is overshadowed by more powerful emotional experiences, such as anger or fear. Primary sadness is not the same as helpless and powerless depression; rather it facilitates acceptance of the reality of loss and moving on.

In Chapter 7, we suggested that anger expression about situations involving abuse is facilitated by active expressive techniques such as empty-chair dialogue. However, it is difficult and possibly inappropriate for clients to express their pain and sadness toward an imagined abusive other, especially one who is unrepentant. Clients are not inclined to be open and weak in front of the perpetrator (Paivio, 1995). Therefore, emotionally focused interventions accessing primary sadness connected with these situations encourage clients to express their pain and sadness to the therapist or a nonabusive other, rather than to an imagined other they do not trust. Markers of emerging sadness at abuse are not good points to initiate imaginal contact with, or encourage active expression to, the abuser. This also is consistent with the adaptive action tendency of sadness, which is one of withdrawal into the self or seeking comfort. Primary sadness is an experience that requires safety, the assurance of succor, and respect for the person's fragility—qualities that are not usually present in the abuser. The sadness is therefore best acknowledged and expressed between the therapist and client, and the client thereby learns to trust and learns an adaptive strategy of seeking comfort from another. It is crucially important for the therapist to be able to respond to that need. The following is an example of accessing pain and sadness associated with sexual abuse.

Client Example

Like many people dealing with the effects of childhood abuse, the client in Chapter 7 who had been molested by his teacher remained angry at the perpetrator. Resolution involved holding the teacher accountable for all the harm he had caused. One of the many things he was angry about was that his first sexual experience was ruined. This was also a source of primary sadness, which the client found more difficult to fully acknowledge. The therapist directed attention to the sub/dominant sadness with responses such as "It's very sad that such a potentially beautiful experience should be tainted with abuse of power and coercion and so much complexity" and "It's such a profound loss." She also *evoked memories* of the loneliness and isolation he had experienced during those years. The secret and shameful relationship had cut him off from friends and family, and he spent his adolescence feeling isolated, alone, dirty, and ashamed rather than happy and carefree.

Evoking memories of the traumatic situations helped him reexperience his "dread" in waiting for the teacher, his attempts to discourage the teacher but ultimate failure and despair, and how truly powerless and innocent he was in those situations. Reexperiencing his childhood innocence helped him later to acknowledge his pain and sadness about his loss and to mobilize compassion for himself, which—along with anger expression—helped to *restructure* or counteract internalized self-blame.

He also had lost close relations with his parents, not only because of the secret which kept him isolated, but because he felt there had been a breach of trust with them. He said, "How could they be so oblivious to what was going on with me, like they chose to bury their heads and not see?" Several sessions during therapy were spent *exploring* bad feelings concerning his relationships with his parents. At expressions of secondary anger, such as the above statement, the therapist reflected the client's "disappointment" that his father was so emotionally absent when he was growing up. Also, at his expressions of irritability at his mother's lack of understanding, the therapist reflected his underlying desire to connect with her. This *accessed* primary sadness that there was so much distance in their relationship; the client wanted to be understood and accepted by his mother. This, in turn, helped motivate renewed efforts to "communicate" with her, to heal their relationship. He reviewed the history of the abuse and *constructed a new narrative* in which neither he nor his parents were to blame, and he held the perpetrator accountable for the harm he had caused.

Client Example

The following transcript is from Session 6 of therapy with another client, "M.," dealing with sexual abuse. It illustrates accessing primary sadness, the close connection between anger and sadness, and the fluid use of empty-chair work for exploration and accessing these different emotions. The client is engaged in a dialogue with her imagined uncle, who had sexually molested her when she was 4 years old. The therapist has just asked her to symbolize what she is angry about:

DIFFERENTIATE FEELINGS

C: (*weepy*) I hate you for making me embarrassed at what I look like . . . unable to give myself to someone without having that image go through my head and just freaking out, never feeling free, always doubting whether they know, or can tell.

T: Like you ruined a part of me and I hate you for that. [Symbolize]

C: Yes, 'cause I can't ever get it back. I'll never know what its like, how my daughter feels about her body ... taken away without my permission or an apology. . . . I hope you're rotting in hell, 'cause you didn't just do it to me but to my sister too, and your own daughter. . . .

T: How dare you do that to us, take away our, my innocence, my self-respect? [Intensify]

C: Yes, how dare you? . . . It was your sickness not ours. (T: Say that again.) It was your sickness not ours. (T: Say it louder.) It was your sickness not ours.

T: How does that feel saying that? [Direct attention]

C: (*weepy*) It feels hard. It's like I don't feel it.

ACCESS PRIMARY SADNESS

T: Feels hard, like it's hard to believe in your words? (C: Yeah.) What *are* you feeling, M.?

C: Just so sad for that little girl (*sobs*) . . .

T: Ah, sad, stay with that, yes, such a huge loss, say more.

C: 'Cause I never felt the same as other little girls . . . (*weeping*) never a moment has gone by when I felt really free and comfortable about myself. It's so unfair—if only I looked right, always feeling there was something wrong with me, or (*pause*) (T: Like what?) feeling dirty.

RESTRUCTURING BY ACCESSING HEALTHY RESOURCES, AND SELF-SOOTHING

T: Ah, yes, feeling dirty, how unfair, how sad that this little girl ends up feeling bad about herself. Can you imagine that little girl here? (*brings empty chair closer, strokes chair*) You, that little girl. What do you want to do or say to her, to yourself as this little girl? [Focus on present, Intensify]

C: (*weeping*) That you're innocent. . . . I wish I could give it all back to you. . . . You deserved to believe you were beautiful.

SUPPORT SELF-AFFIRMING STANCE

T: Yes, a beautiful little girl . . . (*pause; client weeping subsides*) What's happening for you now? [Focus on present]

C: I'm just angry . . . that you (*looks at empty chair*) could have the nerve
    to do that . . . that it was your right, that I was your property and
    you could do what you liked . . . betrayed my trust. . . .

Thus, through memory evocation, painful *primary experience* is
accessed and the client is able to acknowledge the loss of her innocence.
Primary sadness, expressed with the support of the therapist, accesses
healthy resources of self-compassion and self-soothing, and these help
to *restructure* her maladaptive view and experience of herself as dirty.
At the end of the session, the client reports feeling exhausted but, for
the first time in her life, hopeful that she can resolve these issues.

Secondary Sadness or Depression

Depression can sometimes be manifested as uncontrolled expressions
of sadness. People break into uncontrollable tears, against their will, in
response to triggers that the person considers inappropriate and in a
manner that repeatedly interrupts her or his ability to cope.

Feeling hopeless is one of the predominant bad feelings associated
with sadness and distress, and generalized hopelessness is central to
the experience of depression. One of the ways of working with
depression, in an emotionally focused approach, is to heighten awareness of the experience of hopelessness—to help the client sink into and
then explore how that experience is created. The experience of accessing hopelessness in therapy is different from the process of allowing
primary pain. As we have have said, with hopelessness there is less of
a process of "living through" the experience and knowing you can
survive, and more of a remoralization process. This involves overcoming discouragement by accessing internal resources that provide the
desire and courage to carry on. Hope needs to be rekindled, and this
occurs by first facing the hopelessness and fully experiencing it, rather
than avoiding it.

Often, it is difficult for clients to allow themselves to do this
because they spend so much effort trying to stop themselves from
feeling depressed and hopeless. It may seem counterintuitive to experience hopelessness again in therapy, when what they want is to stop
feeling that way. A rationale needs to be provided that clarifies why it
is beneficial to deeply experience one's hopelessness. Examples include
"This is a powerful part of who you are at this time, like it's taking
over. This is the part of you that wants to just give up, sees no point
in going on, sees no meaning or value in life, feels utterly empty. It
makes sense to get to know this part of yourself better, explore it in a
way you can't do on your own, safely, therapeutically. This way, it can

change." Similarly, in working with chronic underregulation of tears, the therapist needs to distinguish between therapeutic weeping and chronic weepiness. Therapeutic weeping involves accessing the primary pain or sadness, and this helps counteract the underregulation of tears that are so close to the surface that they chronically spill over.

In accessing the hopeless state, one also accesses associated emotions such as sadness, fear, or anger, pathogenic beliefs about self and others, unmet wants and needs, as well as fears or perceived barriers to getting needs met. Thus clients will have a better understanding of what is generating their hopelessness, as well as an awareness of their needs as providing healthy resources that can challenge or restructure their hopelessness in therapy. Our clinical experience is that, once hopelessness is deeply felt and explored in the safety of the therapy environment and allowed to run its course rather than avoided, it shifts into a more primary emotional experience. It shifts to acceptance of a specific loss and/or to mobilization of adaptive internal resources. These internal resources—such as unexpressed anger or a desire for contact, or a desire to live and to enjoy life—spontaneously emerge and act as challenges to maladaptive cognitions and feelings of generalized hopelessness.

However, there are contraindications for heightening the experience of hopelessness, such as when clients are feeling suicidal or are at risk for self-harming behavior. In addition, heightening of the intense hostility directed toward the self, which sometimes occur in hopelessness, is counterindicated. These are not productive interventions; rather, intervention at these times needs to center on strategies for regulating the distress and coping with it.

Client Example

The following example illustrates secondary sadness or depression, in which unexpressed primary sadness at loss is the generating condition for the client's depression. It is as though this client was stuck in the depressive stage of grieving rather than moving on to accepting the loss. Moreover, the client's fear of his vulnerability, a process that will be discussed further in Chapter 9, was preventing him from acknowledging his sadness. This man sought therapy for depression precipitated by the end of his marriage. This was complicated by the loss of his job and the immediate need to search for another, which he found difficult to motivate himself to do. The client experienced low energy, poor sleep, weight gain, and withdrawal. He berated himself for his inability to get going and for turning to food for comfort, and attempted to lecture and cajole himself into action. Work in therapy partly involved exploring the conflict between this critical part of himself and his experiencing self—the part of him that was hurt and sad, wanted to withdraw, and needed comfort. Disallowing his sadness and neediness was one of the processes *generating* his depression.

One problem in working with this type of conflict is the difficulty in establishing a collaborative focus on the underlying determinants of the depression. This is because people often align themselves with the critical part of themselves and disavow their internal experience. Thus, this client believed that his hurt and sadness were signs of weakness that were dragging him down and causing his depression, whereas the critical side of himself was helping him to get on with his life. The skill required by the therapist, in these processes, is to validate the values and standards of the critic, the part of him that wants to get on with his life, take care of his health, and be financially secure but, simultaneously, to heighten awareness of the unacknowledged hurts, wants, and needs. Therapy, first, was aimed at helping him become aware of and *explore* how he squashed and rejected that experiencing part of himself and the impact this had on his life. EFT needed to help him see, experientially, that his avoidance was not an effective strategy because it was not alleviating his depression. This would help him accept a *rationale* for getting more in touch with the side of himself that did not want to job search, that wanted to hide away, withdraw, and be taken care of. The therapist suggested that despite, and perhaps because of, his efforts to "whip himself into shape," the hurt and depressed part of him dominated his life. For example, two-chair dialogues between the critical and experiencing parts of himself revealed how strongly the critical part of himself squashed and controlled his experience. Repeatedly, after a few seconds of expressing his feelings of loneliness and defeat, he quickly shifted to lecturing and talking himself out of those feelings. At one such marker, the therapist responded, "It's as if this side [experiencing] of you is not allowed to speak, has no voice. Yet this feeling part is ruling your life, is the most powerful part of yourself, right now. It makes sense to get to know this part of yourself. Try staying with this feeling side a little longer, speak from your sense of hopelessness." It was easy for him to be angry at his ex-wife and about his unemployment, but he seemed to reject his hurt and sadness, despite the fact that he had suffered two major losses and blows to his self-esteem. By focusing on his interruptions of sadness as it emerged in the session, the client came to acknowledge that he did not want to admit that his wife got to him, for then it would be like conceding that she had won. For him, admitting sadness meant admitting failure and defeat. These beliefs now were available for exploration and restructuring.

It is important in these situations to avoid arguments and cajoling clients into feeling their feelings. Overcoming avoidance, in this case, was accomplished first by *validating* and *exploring* his concerns about sinking into hopelessness and sadness and, through empathic responses, repeatedly normalizing and directing his attention to his primary experience and dependency needs. This way he felt safe to let down his guard. Over time, with patience and support, he was able to *access* and fully experience how hurt and sad he was at the loss of his marriage and to acknowledge his feeling of failure. Attention at this point to what he needed led to mobilization of his need for support and connectedness and a sense of his worth as a human being. This, in turn, mobilized internal resources to counteract the depression, and he challenged his maladaptive beliefs about his lack of self-worth from his internal experience. Self-nurturing and self-enhancing behavior and seeking nurturance and support from others followed.

CHAPTER NINE

Fear and Anxiety

*F*ear and anxiety are distinct emotional experiences, although often the terms are used interchangeably. On the one hand, fear is highly unpleasant, with a compelling survival-oriented function—to precipitate one's escape from danger. It is generally a transient response to a specific stimulus that abates after the person escapes from the danger. The intensity of fear responses, degree of arousal to novel stimuli, and vulnerability to panic all vary across individuals and may interact with the presence of interpersonal security.

On the other hand, anxiety is a response to symbolic, psychological, or social situations, rather than immediately present physical danger. Anxiety is a response to uncertainty that arises when the sense of self-integrity, coherence, continuity, or agency is threatened. Certain learning histories characterized by unpredictability and lack of interpersonal control can produce many interpersonal anxieties, including fear of intimacy and fear of losing control. Anxiety also is a key motivator of human action and interaction. The capacity to experience anxiety is almost synonymous with the capacity to plan for the future, and the increased arousal associated with anxiety can enhance performance. Anxiety also can be experienced as excitement depending on how one views the situation. For example, stage fright can either be seen as preparatory excitement or debilitating anxiety. Anxiety is debilitating and dysfunctional when it is intense and chronic, when people are continually anticipating dangers or expecting threats of the past to repeat themselves.

When fear is evoked, action is halted, the environment is vigilantly monitored, and plans for fleeing or avoiding the dangerous situation are made ready. This action tendency is a complex integrated mind/body response. The sympathetic nervous system is aroused, the person feels a rush of adrenaline (epinephrine), becomes more alert, and focuses attention on the immediate situation. Subjective feelings of fear frequently are accompanied by anger, which helps to mobilize the person for strenuous action. Anxiety, on the other hand, results in confusion or in cognitive processes that dominate awareness rather than an explicit action tendency. There is either a diffusion of attention or a narrowing of attentional focus on self. The latter consists of increased arousal and preoccupation with one's ability to perform effectively or to feel safe in the situation.

PROCESS DIAGNOSIS OF DIFFERENT FEAR AND ANXIETY STATES

The complexity of process diagnosis of different fear and anxiety states is illustrated in the following clinical example. A client sought therapy for social avoidance, chronic feelings of loneliness, alienation, and unresolved issues with her parents. Her problems were sufficiently long-standing and pervasive to suggest characterological disturbance. One focus of therapy was the client's ongoing fear of her parents, which stemmed from severe childhood physical abuse from her father and verbal abuse from her mother. Primary fear of her parents thus was originally adaptive because it had helped, somewhat, to keep her out of harm's way. However, it was now maladaptive because it continued to dominate her current relationships with her parents and with others. One marker of such fear occurred in therapy when she recalled a recent experience of visiting her parents and wincing in panic, fearing violence when her elderly father grabbed his walking stick. Appropriate interventions needed to evoke and explore trauma memories in order to restructure maladaptive emotion schemes related to her sense of herself and others formed at the time. Treatment also focused on her generalized anxious avoidance of all close interpersonal contact. She described herself as "buzzing," feeling like there were "klaxons blaring—danger, danger," in interpersonal situations. A core anxious and avoidant emotion scheme, that is, one in which others were viewed as dangerous and to be avoided, was thought to be the underlying determinant of this reaction. Here, immediacy in the therapeutic relationship was an important intervention, and a corrective emotional experience with the therapist was a mechanism of change. Other important interventions promoted allowing and accepting of previously avoided painful emotional experience. She had learned, through parental invalidation and ridicule, to distrust her internal experience, and she had particularly learned to avoid painful experience associated with unmet attachment needs. These expressions of fear in therapy were mixed with sadness and pain and catastrophic expectations about being overwhelmed by her feelings. At such markers, interventions addressed avoidance of pain and disowning of her dependence, weakness, and vulnerability. Finally, memories of parental criticism, ridicule, and beatings, which evoked fear, sadness, and pain, were potentially overwhelming experiences for this client. Therefore, managing anxiety was another aspect of therapy with this client. An appropriate distance from the intensity of experience was established in order to strengthen her sense of control over her emotional experience.

The foregoing example illustrates how assessing which underlying processes are generating the current experience informs intervention. We will not separately discuss process diagnosis of primary adaptive and instrumental fear and anxiety. Most therapeutic work with fear and anxiety involves accessing a complex reaction with maladaptive components and restructuring this maladaptive emotion scheme. This is different from work in emotionally focused therapy (EFT) with primary anger and sadness, which primarily involves accessing adaptive response tendencies. However, it is important to help people acknowledge primary fear, weakness, and vulnerability when they have a facade of strength and ignore their healthy fear or insecurity. It is generally correct to say one works to turn diffuse anxiety into fear of a specific stimulus, internal or external. Just as with other primary emotions, acknowledging primary fear informs one that something is threatening and sets up a task to explore this further, thus enabling the person to access resources to deal with the threat. Instrumental fear, which is designed to avoid responsibility and have others protect one, is recognized and dealt with in much the same way as other instrumental emotions and is rarely the focus of EFT.

Primary Maladaptive Fear

Primary maladaptive fear is like a phobic reaction to thoughts, feelings, and memories, usually associated with traumatic events. Fear was adaptive in the original situation but continues to be inappropriately activated and becomes anxiety. The presence of these processes is identified both by verbal reports of feeling afraid or panicky when nothing is overtly dangerous and by markers of avoidance, such as "I do things to distract myself" or "I try to blot it out of my mind." Reports of intrusive memories of traumatic events—or threatening fantasies or dreams—also can indicate that some core maladaptive fear is operating and needs to be accessed. Most frequently, the person fears reexperiencing the pain and powerlessness of the traumatic event. In these situations the person feels very shaky and in general terms is aware of what it is she or he fears—and is trying to cope with by avoiding dealing with the experience. There are explicit statements of fear as well as physical signs of anxiety in therapy, such as stuttering, shallow breathing, and sighing whenever the trauma-related material is discussed. Alternatively, intense secondary anger reactions can protect against and be a sign of underlying fear. These markers all indicate the need to face the threatening material and deal with it in a safe and validating environment. Treatment involves accessing and exploring complex components of the maladaptive emotion scheme through memory evocation.

Primary Maladaptive Anxiety

Primary anxiety is generated by the activation of a core insecure or vulnerable self-organization or sense of self. Assessment and recognition of this type of primary insecurity in therapy is helped by a knowledge of the person's attachment history, combined with in-session indicators of uncertainty, timidity, hypersensitivity, hypervigilance, and extreme self-consciousness. Markers of intense vulnerability or fragility, associated with this self-organization, occur most vividly in therapy when a client shows anxiety at exposing aspects of self-experience and is guarded or cautious about self-disclosure: "I hate having the spotlight on me."

Pervasively anxious clients are afraid of being judged or misunderstood by the therapist and are not able to disclose their concerns unless they feel safe; such a person is highly vulnerable to abandonment or rejection. This is related to shame-anxiety in which the client anticipates potentially feeling embarrassed, humiliated, or mortified if they reveal core aspects of self-experience, and again this is evident in problems such as social phobia or avoidant personality disorder. The feared or dreaded aspects of self often have to do with neediness, jealousy, or insecurity. Intervention provides the needed safety and empathic affirmation of the threatening core experience to allow self-disclosure. Exploration of the experience follows only after the client feels sufficiently safe and understood.

Sometimes a primary anxious self-organization is indicated by an anxious-avoidant attachment pattern (Bowlby, 1958), as illustrated in the above clinical example. The sense of self has developed from an aversive attachment history so that the person has given up seeking attachment and turned to self-sufficiency. The person's self-sufficiency is accompanied by feeling alienated and alone, and having a limited ability to explore or differentiate internal experience.

In our view the type of maladaptive anxiety that is observed in disturbances such as social phobia is not generated primarily by conscious construals or distorted cognitive appraisals of reality. Rather, such anxiety is generated by a core insecure and vulnerable sense of self that is chronically activated in interpersonal situations. It is this holistic, multicomponent, bodily felt sense of self as ineffective and unprotected that needs therapeutic attention and needs to be changed. Conscious appraisals of the self or situation are by-products of that core self-organization that fuel but do not create the anxiety.

Finally, it is important in working with primary insecurity to recognize the existence of other self-organizations—in particular, to recognize what Winnicott (1965) called the "true self." Clients refer to this as a hidden, essential part of themselves that comprises their adaptive wants and needs. Through negative learning experiences, this part of the self has withdrawn for protection but, in a safe environment, is available as an inner resource. Markers include longing for connection, interdependence, freedom, and spontaneity, as well as the desire to be less cautious and take more risks. Emotionally focused interventions support the emergence of this essential self-organization in fostering the development of a stronger and more secure sense of self.

Secondary Anxiety

How does the therapist identify that certain anxiety is secondary and requires exploration of the underlying determinants rather than working with the anxiety itself? The answer lies in determining the referent of the anxiety. In secondary anxiety it is not the core self that is insecure, like a lost small child in a big world, but rather the person is anxious that an internal experience, such as anger, sadness, or weakness, will threaten the self or an attachment relationship. These experiences are therefore guarded against, leaving the person anxious and vulnerable. It is also useful to distinguish between a core fear of internal experience learned through severely negative attachment experiences and a less central (core) fear of emerging experience stemming from internalized social injunctions such as "Women shouldn't be angry" or "Men shouldn't cry." The former requires considerably more therapeutic safety to access the person's denied core feeling. The latter requires more exploration and questioning of the injunctions, cognitions, or imagined dangers that relate to limited domains of experience.

A special case of avoiding internal experience involves *fear of weakness and disavowal of dependency needs*. This is exemplified by men who react with anger when they feel afraid and needy. Here anger is the end result of a cognitive–affective sequence involving secondary anxiety about primary fear. A related form of secondary anxiety arises in states of confusion and uncertainty about internal experience, or by the inability to label or symbolize internal experience that leaves people disoriented. In these cases, intervention involves experiential awareness training in which the client is helped to attend to a present bodily felt sense, and differentiate and symbolize immediate experience so that it can be integrated into self-experience.

Catastrophic expectations, performance anxiety, and fear of anticipated failure are other common forms of secondary anxiety. Markers of this type of anxiety are future-oriented expectations or imagined dangers, and prototypic "what if?" statements, accompanied by a helpless response, such as worrying about being rejected, failing, or being incompetent. This type of anxiety is generated by maladaptive cognitions and interventions focus on changing the cognitions. In EFT, catastrophic expectations are modified by accessing challenges that emerge from the client's own experience, rather than challenges that come directly from the therapist.

Fear of negative evaluation is another form of secondary performance anxiety. This process involves self-critical cognitions that are attributed to others, such that the person anticipates disapproval and/or rejection. Of course, fears that are based in reality, for example, a gay man who fears homophobic reactions from others, need to be validated, but at the same time hypersensitivity to criticism results from internalized negative self-evaluation. This develops from harsh introjected values and standards, conditional parental acceptance, threats of rejection or disapproval for failure to live up to parental standards, and parental criticism and overcontrol. The person develops a pervasive sense that there is something wrong with him or her that others will find unacceptable. The severity of the original threat plays a central role in the intensity of the fear. For example, a client with a learning disability had been cruelly teased and criticized throughout his years of schooling. As an adult, he continued to be extremely socially avoidant and feared making a fool of himself in social encounters. The generating condition for his current anxiety is his internalized pathogenic belief that he is a "loser." Intervention involved validating the cruelty and painfulness of this learning history but accessing and strengthening his core sense of himself as valuable and needing support.

The above example illustrates another complexity of process diagnosis in this area. It is important to distinguish fear of negative evaluation, which is part of a core self-structure, from more situationally specific secondary anxiety reactions such as speech or performance anxiety. In the latter case, the anxiety may be a function of more easily accessed and modifiable dysfunctional cognitions or imagined dangers. Appropriate intervention here concentrates on teaching present skills to attend to the surrounding world or one's breathing, rather than to worries, and accessing the maladaptive cognitions for change. In the former case, however, the beliefs are part of a more deeply entrenched self-organization involving low self-esteem. Here, intervention focuses more on strengthening the fragile sense of self through empathic attunement and developing self-soothing capacities rather than simply modifying self-statements. (The type of insecurity that is generated by a core sense of self as inferior or worthless will be discussed in Chapter 10 on shame.)

EMOTIONALLY FOCUSED INTERVENTION

Our approach to working with fear and anxiety integrates aspects of other treatment approaches. EFT includes techniques for accessing and modifying maladaptive fear and catastrophic expectations, an emphasis on early attachment relationships and unmet dependency needs, attention to safety, and a curative emotional experience with the therapist, as well as anxiety management strategies when these are appropriate. However, EFT is unique in emphasizing evocation and exploration of the immediate experience of complex fears and anxieties related to the self. We do this for the purpose of exposing these to newly mobilized adaptive primary feelings, needs, and self-soothing capacities that function to modify the fear-producing psychic structures.

Most therapeutic work with fear and anxiety involves helping clients deal with the regulation of underregulated fear. This involves the restructuring of complex maladaptive emotion schemes. Treatment objectives therefore generally differ from those for work with overcontrolled primary anger and sadness. Objectives with fear are to access the core maladaptive fear scheme in order to make the maladaptive aspects amenable to modification. This also differs from work with adaptive fear that involves simply acknowledging the fear and accessing the adaptive action tendency of flight and the need for safety. Accessing the need for safety in both adaptive and maladaptive fear *can* mobilize healthy self-soothing capacities that were not available in the original fear-producing situation. The central problem associated with maladaptive fear and anxiety is that they persist and generalize to current situations where they are no longer appropriate or adaptive. They exist as an overactive alarm system.

Vulnerability of the self is a type of anxiety response that is of particular interest in EFT. This is anxiety that involves the threat of disintegration and fear of the inability to regulate one's own emotions. Feelings of vulnerability come either from fears of abandonment or threat of self and others' condemnation, contempt, or rejection when aspects of self or self-experience are exposed. The action tendency or coping responses include guardedness, covering or protecting the self, and withdrawal and defensive shutting down, so that core parts of the self are not exposed to danger. When this occurs in therapy, treatment involves exposing the vulnerable self both to new experience with the therapist that disconfirms pathogenic beliefs and fears of abandonment, and to a process of self-soothing.

Intervention Principles Applied to Fear and Anxiety

In the following subsections we will discuss intervention principles that are unique to EFT with fear and anxiety. We will not discuss strategies for managing anxiety that are integrated into EFT because these have been well documented in the clinical literature.

Direct Attention to Internal Experience (Bodily Felt Sense)

Helping people focus on bodily experiences related to fear and anxiety is a way of encouraging present rather than future orientation. Here-and-now awareness is an antidote for anticipatory anxiety and "what if" catastrophizing. Helping clients recognize and label anxiety and then symbolize what they are afraid of also reduces anxiety. Finally, attention to internal anxiety-related experience heightens awareness of the powerful effects of anxiety on the body and on cognitive processes. The hypervigilance and self-consciousness of anxiety distracts the person from awareness of other experiences and therapeutic responses can highlight this aspect of fear experience: "Yes, it takes over—hard to attend to anything else, really interferes with your concentration." However, it is inappropriate to focus on bodily sensations if the client is feeling panicky in the session; at such times it is advisable to employ strategies for anxiety management and control, such as regulation of breathing and progressive muscle relaxation.

Intensify Experience

Interventions that intensify experience are intended to heighten aware-ness of unacknowledged threat and access pathogenic beliefs and catastrophic expectations. However, once fear is aroused, one does not generally wish to intensify it. Interventions for therapeutically arousing unacknowledged anxiety include asking clients to exaggerate "fear breathing" (repeated gasps without exhaling), the tension in their shoulders, and their grimaces such that tension builds and is finally released in a flood of tears. Less active interventions include imagining the feared situation and evocative empathic responses that capture the fear experience, such as "I imagine you're really dreading what will happen next," "There's this sense that the rug is gonna be pulled out at any minute," "It's like sitting on a time bomb," or "There's a sense of impending doom . . . how extremely uncomfortable."

A special type of intensification is used to promote client respon-sibility, agency, or sense of control over their experience of anxiety. Clients can be asked to enact how they make themselves afraid, to intensify and exaggerate catastrophizing, thus increasing awareness of agency or how they contribute to their own fear and anxiety. Once the fear is activated, adaptive resources are mobilized in the form of either internally generated challenges to these irrational beliefs or self-sooth-ing responses. This process will be described more fully in the section on therapeutic work with anxiety.

Memory Evocation

Evocation of trauma memories can be stressful and emotionally chal-lenging work for therapists. It can be difficult to hear clients' stories of horror without being disturbed and backing away, rather than helping them approach this material. Nevertheless, this is a crucial intervention principle in working with maladaptive fear related to trauma because clinical and research evidence suggests that reexperi-encing trauma memories in a safe therapeutic environment is the key to changing maladaptive aspects of the memory. Memories of anxiety-provoking or fear-producing situations are evoked, just as they are in work with other primary emotions, through the use of active tech-niques such as enactment, imagery, or systematic evocative unfolding of the situation. These bring alive the memory or relevant fear structure, making maladaptive components available for restructuring in therapy. In the case of trauma, evoking memories is partly for the purposes of exposure and desensitization to avoided aversive stimuli or painful thoughts and feelings. Exposure in EFT is gradual, but not as systematic as in behavioral interventions, and it occurs within an empathic context, rather than explicit skills training. Reexperiencing trauma memories also allows for construction of new meaning in terms of maladaptive perceptions of self, others, and reality formed at the time of the trauma.

Symbolize Experience

Naming what one is afraid of reduces uncertainty, which is the hallmark of anxiety. Once clients symbolize their fear, they can examine the situation and plan to avert potential harm, which increases a sense of control. Moreover, challenges spontaneously emerge while one is symbolizing irrational fears or imagined dangers. Clients are encouraged to specify what is threatening or dangerous with empathic questions such as "There is something threatening or scary about speaking up?" or "It's like something awful might happen if you disagree. Can you get in touch with that feeling—what do you imagine might happen?" Here, catastrophic expectations are "hot cognitions" that emerge from the immediate reexperiencing of fear or anxiety. Clients also need to symbolize their desire to protect themselves against being vulnerable—to armor themselves, put up barricades or walls, or be on guard. Therapists can validate how this feels safe and, if the self-protective strategies are interfering with healthy functioning, also highlight how it separates clients from others and cuts them off.

In situations where avoidance of trauma memories is dysfunctional, symbolizing experience involves helping clients to tell their story in all its detail, to face again the fear, the horror, to uncover the layers of secrets, so these can evolve. Similar interventions with survivors of sexual abuse encourages clients to draw or paint their experiences, the dreaded or shameful situations. This is a kind of exposure therapy, a way of bringing the dreaded material into the open, defusing it, and creating new meaning or narrative about the situation.

THERAPEUTIC EPISODES WITH FEAR AND ANXIETY

Acknowledgement of primary fears, such as fear of abandonment, is part of the ongoing fabric of an empathically oriented, emotion-focused treatment, and we will not concentrate specifically on this. Rather, the specific therapeutic events covered in the subsections below illustrate different intervention strategies for changing the following types of maladaptive fear and anxiety: (1) primary insecure and vulnerable sense of self; (2) primary maladaptive fear related to trauma and abuse;

(3) secondary anxiety about feeling weak and helpless; (4) catastrophic expectations; and (5) secondary performance anxiety or fear of negative evaluation.

Insecure and Vulnerable Sense of Self

An insecure sense of self is rooted in the basic fear that one will be left alone and unable to cope or protect oneself. Such a fear develops from early experiences of actual or threatened loss of attachment and unmet dependency needs. This learned fear can underlie a variety of dependency issues for which people seek treatment, such as agoraphobia, eating disorders, substance abuse, and interpersonal dependency. Clients with these problems seem to lack confidence in their ability to cope and feel desperate because they have difficulty with self-soothing. Therefore, they rely on external supports as a way of managing their fear and insecurity.

Primary insecurity, as a core sense of self that is activated across situations, stems predominantly from inconsistent availability of caretakers, repeated threats of harm, verbal or physical assaults, angry rejection, and neglect. A person with such a learning history responds to actual or threatened loss of attachment with heightened arousal, vigilance, and efforts to control the environment or self, for example, through anger or clinging to the attachment figure in order to avoid or avert anticipated separation. The person learns to view attachment figures as potentially rejecting, abandoning, and hurtful, and the future as uncertain and insecure. The goal of therapy is to strengthen the client's insecure sense of self.

This is accomplished, first, by helping people acknowledge and accurately symbolize their fear of being hurt, left alone, abandoned, or rejected. For example, when clients react with anger or cry in helplessness at rejection, EFT intervention focuses on their underlying experience of fear, which is masked by the secondary reactions. We then explore the multidimensional fear experience in order to access associated needs, pathogenic beliefs, and meanings. Therapist responses highlight and direct client's attention to their internal experience—how they think, feel, act; what they want and need; what is important and meaningful to them. These are the aspects of experience that define the self. One important aspect is the action tendency associated with separation anxiety, which is the primary need for protection from others. Symbolizing this need helps to access healthy resources to get the need met or to develop the adaptive internalized responses for self-soothing. For example, acknowledgement of fear of abandonment can motivate the person to seek needed support from others, including the therapist, or learn to manage without it if the support is not forthcoming. Development of the capacity to look after oneself and rely on one's own resources to get needs met strengthens the sense of self and helps develop confidence that experiences of aloneness are temporary and manageable. The therapeutic relationship provides support while the client explores and engages in such new autonomous behavior. The self is simultaneously strengthened through increased awareness, ownership, and therapist validation of primary wants, needs, and concerns.

EFT interventions for accessing self-related emotion schemes include evocative responding, imagery, or evocation of memories of negative attachment experiences. For example, a client who was afraid of being abandoned and left alone was asked to imagine a specific situation in which she was left alone and to attend to this dreaded experience of aloneness. With the support of the therapist, she was able to deeply experience it, tolerate it, and accept this aspect of herself. Once accepted, her experience spontaneously shifted to imagining ways in which she could cope and take care of herself, by seeking out friends and pleasurable activity. The following example illustrates therapeutic work with this type of primary insecurity.

Client Example

This woman grew up in fear of her father's explosive anger, his physical violence toward her mother, as well as cruel criticisms of her. As an adult, she was timid and insecure, responding to any sign of disapproval or anger the way she had as a child. In these situations, she attempted to "walk on eggshells" in order to prevent the disapproval of others and to stifle her own anger. She then became confused and paralyzed, and ultimately collapsed into numbness, resignation, and depression. She was chronically tense, anxious, felt overly responsible for her family's well-being, and suffered from chronic low self-esteem. These were indicative of a core vulnerable and insecure sense of herself, developed through childhood learning experiences.

One of the client's goals in therapy was to feel less vulnerable in face of her father's ongoing anger and cruel accusations, to feel "not so defenseless in these situations." She added, "Its almost like I can't survive what he dishes out, so I need to have some protection." She also wanted to feel less timid and express herself more freely. She recalled a time when she took a vacation and felt confident, free of anxiety, and truly herself, and she longed to access this strong part of herself more frequently. The therapist *acknowledged* her fear and need for protection, and supported her healthy desire to feel more free and alive. They developed a collaborative *focus* on accessing these healthy internal resources to strengthen her insecure sense of self.

During one session, when the client expressed how she avoided disagreements, didn't want to rock the boat, and couldn't stand up to others, including her father ("like I am not allowed to be who I am"), the therapist asked what frightened her. The client explained that she was afraid of being rejected for speaking her mind, that she was careful not to upset others: "I can't ever be angry—I walk a narrow line, like there are land mines everywhere." The therapist responded, ". . . so careful—somehow if your anger is not contained, something might explode, or. . . ?" This is an example of how therapists can use client metaphors to help *evoke* experience and invite *exploration* of experience with empathic exploratory responses.

Memory evocation also was used to access core emotion schemes with maladaptive beliefs, reactions, construals, and primary emotional experience. The following transcript, from Session 8, illustrates this process. The client has been talking about her chronic tension headaches, which she attributed to excessive responsibility in her family of origin. The therapist has directed her to tell her imagined father about the effects of his parenting on her. In the excerpt below, the client moves in and out of an empty-chair dialogue with her imagined father, turning to the therapist when she needs contact and support. This need for frequent contact with the therapist, during active interventions, is typical of clients who are anxious and insecure. EFT offers all the support that is needed, metaphorically holding the client's hand as they engage in these anxiety-provoking but growth-enhancing activities.

EXPLORE BAD FEELINGS

C: (*speaking to empty chair*) You didn't provide the parenting that I needed or provide an environment that felt safe and comfortable and, because I could see everybody in the family reeling from the way you behaved to them, I took on a parenting role that was way beyond my ability. . . .

ACCESS CORE EMOTION MEMORY

T: This must have been a big strain—see if you can get in touch with any specific memory of any one incident. Can you recall any one time when you were a child. [Memory evocation]

C: I remember I used to sit in the kitchen watching mom getting supper ready, and K. and A. [siblings] were just in diapers, playing on the floor, and I was sitting at the table, in the chair, sitting on my hands, so that I would force myself to be quiet and still and good, and not touch anything I wasn't supposed to touch, or get into trouble . . . and keep K. and A. from getting into trouble, 'cause when you came home from work was when you were very angry, and everything had to be just so, or else you would get angry at everybody, especially mom. So I would try and sit there, and just be perfect and quiet and good, and I remember thinking and watching K., and almost praying, "Don't do this." (T: Praying.) Praying for them to be good, 'cause I knew mom would be the one to get the beating.

T: So somehow I really wanted mom to be spared. [Establish need]

C: But the funny thing is it never worked, because every night, aahh, it would always be the same, but I kept trying.

T: So it never worked but I kept at it, hoping that some way I could make a difference or change . . .

C: And I expended all this energy, did all this stuff with you in mind, that you were going to come home and be angry at us. Every action was always with you in mind, that we had to be a certain way so you wouldn't fly into a rage.

ACCESS PRIMARY INSECURE EMOTION SCHEME

T: So what do you feel as you think about that, that everything was focused on him, on how not to get him angry? [Direct attention]

C: It wasn't fair, it wasn't right. . . . I think that as a child I never got to just be a kid and have fun, because I had to work so hard trying to be good and perfect all the time—I lost my innocence and spontaneity. . . . I was always watching out, always nervous . . . diligent . . .

T: Such a strain, always afraid of . . . what were you afraid of? [Symbolize]

C: I was afraid of what he was gonna do to my mom, I was afraid of what he was gonna do to me, but I was more afraid of what he was gonna do to my mom.

T: That was your main concern, somehow to protect her, that must have been so difficult, so hard seeing how he treated her, seeing what happened between them.

C: I didn't want to see it. Something would turn off. I would go away inside and just not feel it and just not see it. It would be happening, but I couldn't stand to be there, so I just went deep inside, imagined myself away, that I was in some kind of bad dream, you know, and I would wake up when it was all over. That's all I really remember feeling is just dead inside, and just numbed, and just trying to get away even if it was in my imagination. . . . It was just my way of escaping—I could be there but just not see anything or feel anything, just be there but not be there. When it was over, I could just pretend it didn't happen.

T: So somehow that's how I protected myself from feeling too much. [Establish need]

C: Yeah, of course today that happens to me sometimes when people start getting angry around me, and I don't really want to be doing that anymore but . . .

T: No, that doesn't serve you well anymore. See if you can get in touch with one of those bad dream experiences as a child, with the feelings you had during one of those experiences, and speak to your father. [Establish intentions, Refocus attention, Evoke memory]

C: Well, I know that I really hated you when you were hurting mommy. (T: Right.) I used to ask God to take you away.

ACCESS CORE DYSFUNCTIONAL BELIEFS, PRIMARY EMOTION, AND NEEDS

T: Stay with that feeling, say this again, that I hated what was going on, I hated what you did to us. [Intensify]

C: When you were hurting mom, I would say to myself, "I hate you" over and over again, and I would wish all kinds of things would happen to you, and I would focus on . . .

T: Tell him what you would wish.

C: Aahh, I would wish you would die, wish you would be killed, and hurt really badly and, aahh, . . .

T: What are you experiencing as you say this, what's going on for you? You kind of bit your lip and . . . [Focus on present]

C: (pause) Well, I think every time I said these things something else inside would realize that I couldn't do that, I couldn't wish those things and I would just sort of . . . it was a conflict I couldn't handle, so I just kind of . . .

T: Yes, such a conflict for a child, but somehow just wishing that he would just disappear, go away, something would happen that we wouldn't have to deal with you. What else did you wish? [Refocus attention, Establish need]

C: I wished that I could die, and I wouldn't have to feel pain, and I wouldn't have to be saying how much I hate my father. I would rather die than continue that.

T: How hard, as a little girl, to feel this hatred toward your father, so much so that you wished you didn't have to feel it at all.

C: I felt, I just remember feeling sick inside, and felt very bad, felt like I was very bad.

RESTRUCTURE

T: See if you can get in touch with what it was like as that 5-year-old—try changing past tense to present, how I feel terrible inside. [Evoke memory, Focus on present]

C: (*pause; "little girl" tone of voice*) I feel sick inside, I feel all . . . I don't want to be here, and I don't want you to hurt mommy any more.

T: So just let her be, stop this, let her be. [Establish need]

C: I want you to go away and leave us alone, so we can be happy.

T: Say this again. [Intensify]

C: I want you to go away, I want you to leave us alone and go away and never come back, and disappear and never come back, (T: Just leave us alone.) and then we could be happy and mommy wouldn't have to be hurt all the time, and I could be happy and be a little girl again—safe.

SUPPORT EMERGENCE OF STRONGER SELF

T: Right, I want to be happy and free, just get away from us. How are you feeling now? [Direct attention]

C: I just want you to go away and not come back, we all hate you, and I don't care if we're poor, we'd just be so happy, aahh (*weeps*), I just can't say any more.

T: How does it feel to have said that? [Direct attention]

C: I dunno, aahh, I feel very sad, a little nervous and scared, but I just feel mostly sad . . . to feel this way toward my father, and also mad. I needed a good father. None of us deserved what we got. He was bad really bad.

The client goes on to explain that she has never said these things before and, although it's painful, she believes it is important to acknowledge her childhood experience. The above transcript also illustrates the relationship between anxiety and depression generated by a core self-organization (Paivio & Greenberg, 1997). Reexperiencing her core insecurity also accessed her weak/bad sense of self, formed in childhood, that is a major generating condition for her chronic depression. As a child, she repeatedly felt weak because she was powerless to change the family situation despite her desperate efforts, and she felt bad for hating her own father. When the client and therapist later processed the whole experience more fully, it was her healthy distrust and desire for distance from her abusive father, rather than her fear and acting as the dutiful daughter, that the therapist supported. The intervention had accessed her anger-based, adult resources to set boundaries and protect herself, and these feelings were used to *restructure* the insecure/vulnerable emotion scheme.

An important aspect of therapy with this client was also mobilizing her self-soothing capacities to strengthen healthy self-regulation. It is important in EFT, as in other therapy approaches, to determine the coping resources and skills that clients have to draw on, and utilize these in therapy. The therapist was aware of this client's strengths, and when markers of competence and strength emerged, she directed the client to attend to those experiences, thus supporting the emergence of healthy resources. For example, when the client recalled a holiday trip when she felt free and alive, the therapist *acknowledged* her longing to access this part of herself more often and asked her to attend to her internal experience as she recalled that situation. During another session, the client recalled a recent incident of feeling panicky at her father's angry accusations, over the phone, and how she felt like a "fragile little girl." The therapist asked the client, "What do you say, how can you calm and take care of the fragile little girl?" The client asserted that she didn't deserve his unwarranted anger, and the therapist supported her standing up for herself by suggesting, "Imagine confronting your father, only speak to him with your stronger self at your side—what do you want to say from that protected stance?" This intervention supported the *mobilization* of her stronger voice and healthy self. The client said to her imagined father, "I am not for your use, you don't own me." The therapist intensified her experience by asking her to say it again and to check how it felt on the inside. This strategy for accessing internal resources was utilized again when the client experienced anxiety at the impending termination of treatment.

Primary Maladaptive Fear Related to Trauma and Abuse

Traumatic events involve fear for one's own or others' physical integrity, accompanied by feelings of profound helplessness. Such events can produce changes in memory, cognition, emotion, and physiological arousal and lead to a disruption of the capacity for integrated and coordinated functioning (Janoff-Bulman, 1992; Herman, 1992). Fundamental assumptions about oneself and the world are shattered, maladaptive beliefs about self and others are formed, and the capacity for self-soothing and calming breaks down. Posttraumatic stress disorder (American Psychiatric Association, 1994) is a problem state that consists of three classes of symptoms: (1) hyperarousal and alertness for danger; (2) intrusive memories, thoughts, and feelings associated with the trauma; and (3) avoidance of reminders of the trauma, including detachment or numbing of feeling.

Profound helplessness seems to be the core damaging experience of trauma, and restoration of a sense of power and mastery are central to recovery. Intrusive memories and reexperiencing the trauma, in thought, dreams, and even in action, appear to be attempts to undo the traumatic experience and to rework the material in order to assimilate it into existing representations of reality. However, the experience is so painful that people dread and avoid it as much as possible, thus perpetuating the symptoms.

EFT for maladaptive fear stemming from trauma and abuse involves exposure to avoided emotional memories or experience associated with the trauma. The fear structure is accessed, for example, through imagery and enactments, and dreaded internal experience is faced and changed by accessing new and adaptive information. Again, the process of exposure in EFT is implicit in the process of exploration, rather than explicitly structured *in vivo* exposure or systematic desensitization.

Clients with disturbances related to posttraumatic stress disorder are encouraged to disclose details of the trauma, that is, symbolize the meaning of the traumatic experience by telling their story. This includes their sense of dread, what they were afraid of, how feelings of powerlessness immobilized them or made them unable to concentrate or think clearly, as well as the meanings and beliefs formed or shattered through the trauma. These are made available for exploration and collaborative construction of new meaning in therapy. Helping the person overcome maladaptive avoidance of memories and painful experience is facilitated by repeated evoking and exposure at a tolerable pace and by expression of anger and sadness. Anger, in particular, is self-empowering and counteracts the powerlessness of fear. However,

anger at abuse, without reexperiencing the fear, will not be as therapeutic. In order for change to occur, the fear structure has to be
accessed, such that the fear is actually experienced. In this way, new
experiences and information can be integrated into the fear structure
and reprocessing can take place. Importantly, the therapist's calming
presence provides a new interpersonal experience to facilitate both
accessing and reprocessing fear.

   Although EFT intervention accesses emotion memories at a safe
pace, disclosure and reexperiencing of traumatic events in therapy is
painful and can evoke intense anxiety. Therefore, clients' capacity to
tolerate reexperiencing such events and to manage anxiety, both in the
session and outside of therapy, is carefully monitored. EFT emphasizes
and supports clients' agency and sense of control over their experience.
Clients are encouraged to set their own pace, to use whatever internal
resources they have to distance themselves from potentially overwhelming experience. For example, well-learned avoidance strategies are
framed as skills that the clients also can use to control arousal levels.
The client's sense of control over the therapy process is essential for
someone whose problems stem from experiences of profound powerlessness and loss of control, and collaboration on the goals and tasks
of therapy is critical in work with issues of trauma and abuse (Paivio
et al., 1996). The following client example illustrates managing client
anxiety while accessing trauma memories.

Client Example

One aspect of therapy with this client was presented in Chapter 7 on
anger. She sought therapy to resolve issues stemming from the suicide
of her mother when she was 10 years old. Her symptoms were
consistent with a diagnosis of posttraumatic stress disorder and included intrusive memories and dreams, chronic anxiety, hypervigilance, and irritability, as well as avoidance of situations and memories
of the trauma. In therapy, the shift in her experience took place
through repeated exposure to painful memories and experiences, by
accessing meanings and beliefs formed at the time of the trauma, and
by fully experiencing and expressing her anger and sadness at the
profound losses she had experienced. Here, we will focus on accessing
and restructuring maladaptive fear and avoidance of trauma memories.

   At the beginning of therapy, the therapist *acknowledged* how painful
and difficult it was for the client to face this material. However, they
agreed that making peace with her mother's death and no longer being
tormented by it would require facing the painful, dreaded memories
from the past. They established this as the *focus* for therapy. Thus

chronic avoidance was validated as a strategy that had helped her cope in the past, but it was also recognized as one of the *underlying determinants* of her ongoing distress and turmoil. The primary intervention for helping this client work through these issues was empty-chair dialogue with her imagined mother.

Once a supportive empathic bond was established, the client was asked to imagine her mother in the empty chair. This first encounter powerfully *evoked* memories of the traumatic event of finding her mother dead. In reexperiencing her horror, the client had difficulty breathing and her voice caught in her throat. The therapist monitored her ability to tolerate this experience and helped her manage her anxiety as she described the scene. Thus the therapist provided safety and supported her need for control over the experience. The following transcript is from Session 3, in which the client first confronts memories of the trauma. The excerpt begins after the client has related a recent family crisis that evoked resentment about her mother's absence:

ACKNOWLEDGE AND EVOKE PAINFUL EXPERIENCE

C: I feel angry and a bit shortchanged . . . that she should have been there for many things in our lives and this, uhh, this is another situation where I feel, I've felt like this many times in my life, but I feel very much like that.

T: Yeah, I can see it in your face, you know "I wish you were here" and I really feel . . . I wonder if you could imagine talking with your mother, if we put her in this chair, and say those things to her . . . would you be able to do that? [Focus on present]

C: (*laugh*) I hope nobody is watching this, I feel like a real cuckoo bird (*laugh*).

T: (*laugh*) Well, one of the neat things about therapy is that you get to do loony things that you don't get to do outside.

C: Interestingly enough, I do talk to her sometimes.

ACCESS CORE EMOTION MEMORY

T: You do? (C: Oh, yeah.) Well, that's great, M. OK, so can you, that sounds like, if it's something that you do ordinarily, it makes even more sense. Can you imagine her sitting there? What does she . . . make contact with her . . . what does she look like to you? How do you see her? [Direct attention]

C: (*clutching at her collar, shallow breathing*) You know the image that is most . . . my first image of my mother is after she died, that is the first thing that I see.

T: It's OK, so can you tell me, what do you see? I know it's painful, but it may be helpful to say. [Focus on present]

C: (*crying*) There are two things, the first, the first, I, in my mind, is when, when, when she was actually in the coffin (*crying*) . . . sorry (*sobbing*) . . .

T: That's alright, yes, I know.

C: She was laying in the coffin and . . . that's the first image I have of my mother, that's, that's the first one (*sobbing*). The second one is the blood and the mess when I found her because . . .

T: Oh, yes, how horrible.

C: . . . and that helplessness of trying to shake her awake, like it was a bad dream (*sobbing*).

T: Just the horror of it all, like this really couldn't be happening. . . . Make it all go away. [Symbolize, Express empathic affirmation]

C: She can't be dead (*sobbing*) . . . and then, and then, I've tried to see her as I remember her and through pictures. I don't even know if it's a photograph or my own recollection, I honestly don't know, (T: right.) I don't know.

T: Yeah, how sad, you try to see her and there is some sense that these other powerful images block out your own memories of the way she was. Those horrors are what's in the forefront.

C: (*crying*) And I have, that very much bothers me, I cannot, um, um, other family members, or there's been a funeral to attend, I have a very very difficult time, I can't go to a wake, I cannot look at a body, I don't want to go anywhere near a coffin, (T: OK.) I'm terrified, (T: Yeah.) I can't, and I have difficulty with that . . . I can't, I can't (*sobbing*).

T: So any of those situations just bring up the whole horror of . . .

C: I see her and she is . . . it is just very very very upsetting.

T: Yeah, yeah, I can well imagine, I mean I can *only* imagine, and I know how painful this must be for you, but when you talk, you said you talk to your mother sometimes, you have conversations with her, how do you imagine her then? [Promote control, Refocus attention]

C: (*crying*) I think, I don't even think, I guess I don't imagine her, I just talk to her, it's like talking to yourself, it's sort of . . . talking into space, like you might pray or talk to God or something. When I think about God, I don't have an image of God. When I go to church, in my mind, I'm just, I just think He hears me.

T: So there is this, for your mother, when you speak with her there is just this amorphous presence, there's not really . . .

C: Yeah, there's not, there's not an image when I'm going on like that, and I'm usually angry when I do that.

T: Uh-huh, I mean I'm wondering if there is a way we can do that here, I mean if you could sort of talk to that chair, and have it be blank rather than . . . and just, you could start out by even saying that, you know, mom, you're just kinda this amorphous presence. The images I do conjure up are unbearable, so I'm just going to put a blank space there—could you do that? Carry on a conversation that way? Or anyway you can. [Evoke memory]

C: I find it difficult. (T: Alright.) Again, that's something you do in your private times. I feel a little silly, I have to admit, I feel a little silly, um—it's if I'm very angry or upset, and I find after I'm able to say it, I do calm down, it's not upsetting me as much usually when I can say it, that is how I feel, and even as recent as last night I'm thinking, mom, why aren't you here? Why can't you (T: OK.) be here to deal with these things? (T: OK, OK, OK.) You know, you have really let a lot of people down.

EVOKE EXPERIENCE

T: Good, that's good, what you're saying, and it seems important to imagine expressing it directly to her. And, if you like, we can just imagine her here as you normally do—I think that there is value in that. So, mom, you should be here!

C: (*crying*) You should be here. Why did you hurt me so much? Why did you do what you did? It was really selfish.

T: It was incredibly selfish of you to leave us alone.

C: And I feel cheated, I feel you cheated me out of a lot of things in life, a lot of my joys and sorrows, that I wanted someone to share with, and you weren't here.

ACCESS PRIMARY ANGER AND SHAME

T: So you cheated me, out of a mother. I'm angry at you for that. [Promote agency, Intensify]

C: Yeah, I'm really angry at you for that, really angry (*sobbing*).

T: Good, that's really good, breathe as you say this. "Damn you"—what happens as you say this—"I'm angry at you"? Breathe, keep breathing, that's good, what happens as you say those things to your mother? [Focus on present, Promote client sense of control, Direct attention]

C: I feel a bit relieved . . . I feel I do need to say those things to her, I feel like . . . look this is how I feel, it is inexcusable, and everybody has made excuses for you for a long time and . . . I realize that life has to go on, I think for the most part I have gone on with my life, it's not, it's time to admit that it was an atrocity and it wasn't right . . . and this is the reality of it. . . .

PROMOTE CLIENT SENSE OF CONTROL OVER EXPERIENCE

T: Right, and you need to give voice to this reality. . . . I'm wondering, I mean I was so aware of you almost not breathing as you were doing it, yeah, very very hard, yeah, so its important to breathe through it. [Focus on present]

C: It was very difficult.

T: And for me, I want to, I mean, I believe absolutely that it is important that you give voice to these things, and I don't want to push you, I want to encourage you, but I want you to set your own limits and set your own pace, and so engage in the task when you can and to pull yourself out of it when you need to. So you, in a way, have to guide me in that respect—does that make sense? 'Cause I want to encourage but I don't want to push you. I want you to go only where you feel safe to go. . . . This is just a tool, this is just a way of helping you, huh, get in touch with some feelings and some pain that I think have been sitting like this great lump, for a long time. And if you felt a little bit of relief in terms of saying just this little beginning, then there is potential for a much greater sense of relief, I think.

C: I do feel a little relieved. . . . I think, when you say you don't know how far to push me, I think that that was the ultimate sore spot, and that is the ultimate sore spot for me . . . but I'll have to find a way of dealing with things, like my image of her, that bothers me, 'cause it frightens me (T: Yeah, yeah.) . . . and I have recurring nightmares that I've had since I was a child, and that nightmare is just that . . . (*relates dream*) . . . and it's horrifying to me, it really

really frightens me, and when I'm dreaming I know that, I know it's coming and I'm trying to tell myself, "Wake up," in my dream, (T: Right.) because it is the same one all the time.

T: Right, so stop, I don't want to feel this again.

The therapist encourages the client to keep breathing and to recall the details of finding her mother, helps her reexperience the trauma scene, then validates her experience, by saying, "Yeah, such incredible turmoil and chaos and things spinning out of control, your whole life out of control, really."

Continued *exploration* and *evocation* focused on facilitating a sense of control for the client over this dreadful experience. Dialogue with the mother without imagining anything concrete but just a sense of her mother's "presence" was a kind of gradual exposure that helped the client manage her anxiety while she accessed painful experience. Gradually she was able to tolerate the experience and reported needing to "talk" to her mother. Therapy, however, did trigger an increase in the client's anxiety, and this required monitoring both in therapy and between sessions. Each session began by checking the client's state during the preceding week and ended with talking about how she could cope during the coming week. Dialogues and memory-evocation interventions were interspersed with exploration of ongoing life problems to help the client tolerate or manage the intensity of reexperiencing.

A critical moment, near the end of therapy, involved articulating a core pathogenic *belief* related to her insecurity that perhaps she had never been loved. This exemplifies how the trauma had shattered or cast doubt on her fundamental childhood assumptions. The client stated that, despite the family chaos, she had always felt loved as a child but since the trauma she had begun to doubt her perceptions. The therapist asked her to express this doubt and her insecurity to her imagined mother. This intervention *evoked* other memories of her childhood, including positive and nurturing experiences with her mother. It helped bring alive poignant memories of her mother as warm and nurturing, and the therapist directed her attention to her internal experience of these memories. She reexperienced the warmth and nurturing she had received as a child from her mother, and said, "I feel good, warm and secure, for the first time since your death. I want to remember this and feel more of this." Thus, reexperiencing positive memories helped disconfirm her pathogenic belief, *restructure* her core insecurity, and *construct new meaning* surrounding her childhood and her mother's death. The therapist *acknowledged* and validated the emergence of self-affirmation and the view that, despite her desperate act, her mother had loved her.

Secondary Anxiety

There are various types of secondary anxiety, and in all such cases the anxiety is secondary to some other cognitive and/or core emotional process. We will later illustrate intervention for exploring catastrophic expectations, and therapeutic work with performance anxiety and fear of negative evaluation. First, we will briefly discuss anxiety about feeling weak and helpless.

Fear of Feeling Weak and Helpless

One experience that particularly makes people feel anxious is the feeling of dependence and weakness. Socialized fear of weakness is frequently observed in men, but it also is observed in women who have been socialized to be competent in caring for others rather than receiving care. They have been rewarded for nurturing others, for being strong and "put together" themselves, and therefore may disavow dependency needs and be fearful of asking for help, of feeling weak and needy. Feeling anxious and afraid in some manner repeats childhood feelings of helplessness and, for some people, is inconsistent with a competent view of themselves. However, feeling weak, vulnerable, and fearful in response to stressful life events is not childish but human.

Therapy aims at helping clients overcome defenses and express their neediness. Similarly, cultural injunctions against men crying or showing signs of weakness leads to them needing to be strong and in control, and to anxiety about feelings of powerlessness or vulnerability. Some men who disavow dependency needs and, at the same time, have a fear of abandonment may well turn to anger and brutality in an attempt to avoid abandonment.

Anxiety about dependence stems from internalized injunctions and/or from a type of conditioned anxiety from early experiences of being hurt, disappointed, or betrayed, rather than being cared for, during times of neediness and vulnerability. People learn to disavow dependency needs because frustration of these needs was too painful. Therapy helps people overcome secondary emotional reactions and defenses, such as denial and anger that protect against feeling weakness and dependency. Mechanisms of change in therapy involve overcoming fear and avoidance, and allowing and accepting the warded-off experience of primary weakness and insecurity, as a healthy aspect of self and an inevitable part of being human. This is achieved by exploring the avoidance process and the internalized messages against feelings. Intervention strategies for overcoming avoidance of weakness are similar to those for overcoming avoidance of other primary emotions except that the relationship with the therapist often plays a more central role in overcoming fear of weakness. Trust needs to be developed before the client can reveal and acknowledge his or her neediness to the therapist, and empathic affirmation of vulnerability and responsiveness to client disclosure are important interventions.

Catastrophic Expectations

This type of secondary anxiety can be similar to fear of internal experience, discussed earlier, when clients catastrophize about their feelings. Anxiety is generated by maladaptive anticipating processes in which clients imagine specific anxiety-provoking situations and dreaded outcomes. Here a fear of failure in some specific performance is the source of anxiety, rather than a core insecure self-organization. Sometimes negative expectations and anticipations about circumscribed events, however, stem from a core anxious and vulnerable sense of self. In these cases, working with this core sense of self becomes important.

Catastrophic expectations also can stop people from pursuing what they want or value. In these situations, anxiety is secondary to the imagined harms or negative consequences and, again, these negative outcomes threaten self-esteem or security. Intervention consists of heightening clients' awareness of what they are doing to themselves—in this case, scaring themselves. Clients' agency in the process and awareness of how they contribute to creating their experience of anxiety is highlighted, along with specifying the irrational beliefs or catastrophic expectations that generate the anxiety. Internally generated challenges to these expectations are then accessed from basic needs and concerns, the part of self that wants to engage and explore.

One intervention we have found particularly effective is two-chair enactment, in which the client directs specific catastrophizing statements at another part of themselves in another chair. They articulate imagined dangers, such as "I will be put down", "make a fool of myself", or "go crazy" and this heightens awareness of the fear-producing process. Clients are encouraged to exaggerate these statements ("Say it again"; "Do it some more"; "Tell him what else he should be afraid of") in order to intensify experience and feel the impact of such statements. This activates the anxiety response. The therapist helps symbolize the process with responses, such as "This is how you scare yourself" or "This is how you stop yourself from feeling?"

After one or several repetitions, a shift occurs. Clients experience themselves as agents in contributing to their anxiety reactions. An observational stance arises in which clients disembed from feeling anxious and can see how their thoughts produce their anxiety. Mastery needs are then mobilized and used to access internal resources and self-soothing capacities that challenge the fear-producing cognitions and help calm the self. Thus, clients can learn to comfort themselves, challenge their maladaptive self-statements or beliefs, as well as become experientially aware of how they are agents in creating their own fear experience. This is empowering and increases feelings of self-control. It is as if, in externalizing and making explicit the catastrophizing cognitions, the client sees them clearly for the first time, is able to examine how realistic or unrealistic they are, and spontaneously challenges unrealistic statements. This differs from a cognitive approach because the therapist does not directly challenge clients' beliefs by asking questions about supporting evidence, but rather directs clients to attend to their internal experience in order to access the adaptive needs. Restructuring occurs when the growth tendency, healthy adaptive resources, and alternate goals and needs are accessed as part of the multilevel emotion scheme that is activated. With the therapist's support, these healthy needs act as challenges to anxiety-producing cognitions.

Clients who have difficulty self-soothing or managing arousal and fear may need to be taught self-soothing skills in conjunction with experiential awareness. Clients also are taught, implicitly and explicitly, to attend to what is occurring in the present, rather than anticipating the future, thus helping to counteract anticipatory anxiety.

Client Example

This client (discussed earlier in Chapter 8 on sadness and distress) was abandoned by her husband and was afraid of getting involved in another intimate relationship, even though she longed for companionship. The following transcript illustrates exploration of her conflict and learned fear of intimacy, accessing maladaptive cognitions, and the resolution and restructuring of these beliefs.

C: I'm terrified, (T: Mm-humm.) I'm terrified to even think of taking a chance like that.

T: So that would almost be too much to bear, to be let down again.

C: No, I just don't think I could take it, to tell you the truth, I don't think I could. . . . Part of me says I would just rather be on my own, and come and go as I please but, huh, part of me says I would like to share with someone. I can see one being terrified of imminent danger, fear of someone hurting them, that type of thing, but I'm so terrified of this, I don't know.

FOCUS ON DETERMINANTS

T: So what's the fear, what's the danger for you? [Symbolize]

C: Being hurt. . . . Emotionally it was painful, not physically but emotionally.

T: Emotionally it was excruciating by the sounds of it. . . . So one important way it impacts your life, it seems, is in terms of getting involved in other relationships. [Symbolize]

C: Yes, because I think I didn't get caring and the love and the affection—the emotional needs met—from the person I really cared about, and this was the person I was the most vulnerable with. I allowed for him to know how I really felt, at least I really thought I did.

T: So you allowed yourself to get really close and he hurt you. . . . It seems, in terms of your current, um, situation, that there is part of you, it is almost as if there are two sides of you. One side is saying, "Gee, I would really like to get involved, I would really like to have a companion, someone close." And there's another side saying, "I couldn't stand the thought." This other part is saying, "No, danger, don't."

C: Yeah, but you know, when I do get into the relationship, I'm the one that is frightened by it, I'm the one that deliberately does something to pull away, it's not the other person.

EXPLORE FEAR-PRODUCING PROCESS IN TWO-CHAIR DIALOGUE

T: So it sounds like you're saying, "Danger, danger," that part of you that is saying, "Danger, back off, don't get too close," takes over and ends up ending the relationship. . . . That sounds incredibly important, I mean, that sounds like, um, a powerful part of your personality right now. . . . We could spend some time exploring those two parts of yourself, the part of you that is saying, "It's too scary," and the part that says, "But I want to, I want to get involved, I want to be close." (C: OK.) What we'll do is put the part of you that is saying all the dangers over here, in this chair, and really speak to this other part of yourself. So it's like two parts of yourself. Just tell her, this other part of yourself, why she shouldn't get involved, what she should . . . [Promote agency]

C: You know, I've actually done that to myself, I've actually said, "OK, now this is a nice person, um, just take it easy and let things happen and don't get scared and run."

Access Maladaptive Cognitions

T: So that's the other part. Here, from this chair, tell her what will happen, what she *should* be afraid of . . . (*pause*), all the reasons she shouldn't get involved . . . (*pause*) "He'll hurt you." [Symbolize]

C: He'll hurt you by not, um, showing up. He'll, um, say something, he'll do something and he won't, and you can't depend on that person to do something, and he won't be there for you, he'll just not show up, or not call, or not . . .

T: So he will let you down. [Symbolize]

C: And he'll let you down and you've been let down too many times, so don't let it happen again, because it will happen . . . mm-humm, it will happen, so just don't get into the relationship to the point where you've allowed that person to take over . . . because they always take over! And then you lose yourself.

T: So it's kinda like I'm afraid for you, I need to protect you.

C: Mm-humm, I am, I'm afraid to let my guard down. . . . No, I won't, I won't let you get involved.

T: Can you come over here (*points to other chair*)—so I wonder what happens as you hear that "I won't let you get involved." [Promote agency]

C: (*switches chairs*) But I'd like to get involved,

Restructure by Accessing Primary Wants and Needs in Order to Challenge Maladaptive Beliefs

T: Can you tell her some of the things that you would like, what it is that you want?

C: I'd like to have somebody to share dinners with, share holidays with . . . someone caring and sharing, but not totally take over and not allow me to be my own person, because that has always happened.

T: So I want to be my own person, but I also want to share my life. [Establish intentions and needs]

C: But I can't seem to do both. I want to share and yet the other person always seems to take over and, I can't, um, I lose myself.

T: OK, come over here. (C: *Switches chairs.*) That sounds like the other part of you, this warning saying "You can't do that, you can't seem to share your life and not lose yourself, you're going to lose yourself." Is that kinda what you're saying? [Focus on present]

C: Yeah, you're going to lose yourself, if you let them step over the line, then you're not your own person anymore, you're not the person that can come and go and do her own thing. That other person takes over and your things you want to do, you can't do anymore—it's like you choose that type of person, I don't know.

ACCESS CORE MALADAPTIVE EMOTION SCHEME AND MALADAPTIVE BELIEF

T: Maybe you choose? . . .

C: (*crying*) Why have I allowed this? Why have I allowed this? Is it because my need for someone to care about me is so much that I lose myself in the relationship?

T: Somehow it is so important to be needed and wanted, it hurts, there's a lot of pain in there, yeah, yeah, yeah.

C: (*sobbing*) That's why I don't want it. . . . Why would anyone want anything that bad, that hurts to that point? Why do I go back for more? (*pause*) For years and years and years, with my husband, I kept saying, "Oh, he'll change, maybe he'll see he's got a good family, and he'll change," because we didn't do anything that he wouldn't want to be with us.

RESTRUCTURE BY ACCESSING PRIMARY NEED

T: We didn't deserve this, and clinging, clinging to this hope, that he would finally see . . . but somehow at the time it's like, "I can't bear the thought of you leaving me." [Symbolize]

C: Mm-humm, it was devastating, absolutely devastating!

T: So I may not survive, almost this feeling of not being able to survive.

C: I didn't think I was going to get through it, and I didn't have anybody to turn to, I didn't have anybody! I didn't have a soul to talk to.

ACCESS INTERNAL RESOURCES

T: So alone . . . so frightening to be so alone, like you can't bear to go through it again, as if the same thing would happen. [Direct attention, Symbolize]

C: But I did get through it, you know. And, you know, it wouldn't necessarily happen again—I've learned more in the last 20 years than some people do in a lifetime. . . .

SUPPORT SELF-AFFIRMING STANCE

T: Yeah, you're not the same woman you were 20 years ago.

The above transcript also illustrates the relationship between core insecurity formed in adult attachment and secondary fear generated by the client's maladaptive cognitions and catastrophizing. The first phase, working with the fear of getting close, involves accessing the expectations of danger. The last part of the work accesses her maladaptive core scheme of insecurity. Through accessing the core insecure emotion scheme associated with her abandonment, the client then experientially understands and accepts that her fear of being left alone with four little children is what kept her in the relationship. Her current maladaptive beliefs that were formed at the time and contribute to her fear of intimacy are challenged through accessing current resources and the awareness that she is not so vulnerable now. Her perspective shifts from one of dependence to one of coping, from the goal of fearfully protecting herself to a goal of asserting her needs for both companionship and autonomy.

Performance Anxiety and Fear of Negative Evaluation

Performance anxiety can be the result of negative evaluations of self which are attributed to others and thus are generated by internalized self-criticisms and harsh judgments, resulting in fear that one will be judged harshly and rejected. Performance anxiety, therefore, is viewed as a secondary anxiety process, secondary to the operation of a self-critical self-organization. This is closely related to the processes involved in low self-esteem and shame, which will be discussed in Chapter 10. Therapy aims at helping the client articulate the imagined negative or critical views of others and gradually understand these as coming from internalized views of the self. The point here is that the negative cognitions that result from a more fundamental emotion scheme can often be changed by bringing them to awareness and mobilizing an internal challenge. At times, however, this is insufficient and the core scheme has to be worked on.

Performance anxiety also can be associated with fear of the therapist's negative evaluation, and for this reason socially anxious clients often find it difficult to engage in active interventions in therapy. Trust and safety in the therapeutic relationship, established over time, are critical aspects of the therapy process. Immediacy in exploring anxiety and feared judgments from the therapist is an important intervention strategy. The following client example illustrates this type of therapy with a client who is highly socially anxious. It illustrates the relationship between catastrophic expectations about internal experience, fear of negative evaluation by the therapist, and performance anxiety that interferes with exploration using the two-chair dialogue intervention.

Client Example

This man came to therapy with "stress" and chronic anxiety, which prevented him from returning to work, and unresolved feelings of hurt and anger from his childhood. He had recently completed a treatment program for drug abuse and had been "clean" for 10 months. He described himself as having "codependency" problems, being a "people pleaser," and dealing with conflict by staying out of the way. This was how he had learned to cope with an abusive and highly critical stepfather, and this was how he coped with an abusive employer in his last job. He was chronically anxious and insecure, had low self-esteem, and feelings of inferiority and worthlessness. He also felt blocked and unable to express his feelings, and his anxiety in early therapy sessions was obvious. He had difficulty breathing, beads of sweat broke out on his forehead, and he became easily confused, especially when asked questions about his internal experience. He said his mind was "racing." He expressed discomfort with the lack of structure at the beginning of sessions. In *exploring* these bad feelings, he said that he felt pressure to say the right thing, wondered what the therapist was thinking about him, and ended up "blabbering about nothing" just to fill up the silence. The therapist *acknowledged* his discomfort, and together they *collaborated* on what was the best way to proceed. They agreed that, as much as possible, she would structure and take the lead at the beginning of sessions by suggesting a specific focus rather than leaving it open ended. This helped him disclose further that trust was difficult for him, that he feared judgment and evaluation, and they agreed that one of the goals of therapy was to develop trust and that this would probably develop slowly. Another goal was to help him become emotionally unblocked—first by exploring what was keeping him blocked and unable to access his feelings.

He described himself as wanting to "let it out," although he did not know what "it" was, and at the same time holding back, experiencing constriction and pressure in his chest. The therapist *acknowledged* his struggle, "like having your foot on the gas and the break at the same time," and suggested they try using the two-chair dialogue intervention to *explore* this process and understand it better, to clarify these two parts of himself. When the client said the intervention made sense, but he felt "stupid" talking to himself, the therapist again collaborated with him concerning the task in order to reduce his performance anxiety. She responded, "We don't have to use the chairs—that's just a tool to help us clarify the two parts of yourself, to keep them really separate so we understand them better. But if it interferes, if it's not helpful, there's no point. I just think its often very helpful and worth a try. If it's not helpful, we'll do something else. Are you willing to give it a shot anyway, and see what happens?" They agreed that the client would switch back and forth between the two chairs to clarify the two parts of himself, but he would speak with the therapist rather than carry on a dialogue with himself. This provided the support he needed and reduced his performance anxiety, his concern about feeling "stupid" talking to himself.

The process of *exploring* his struggle and conflict became one of specifying what was threatening about his feelings. While he was in the "controlling" chair, the therapist empathically conjectured that there was something about his emotions he didn't quite trust. She asked what he imagined would happen if he got in touch with his feelings. This *accessed* maladaptive cognitions that were a combination of catastrophic expectations about being overwhelmed, "a puddle on the floor," and fear of being negatively evaluated by the therapist—again, looking "stupid" for losing control, not "doing it right." Articulating these beliefs quickly evoked the other side of himself, the side that said, "But I have to get it out." These were the core experience and needs that acted to *challenge* his maladaptive cognitions. At this marker, the therapist directed him to switch to the experiencing chair and speak from the part of himself that wanted to relax control: "There's something very important about that. What's important about expressing your feelings?" He said he wanted to feel free and feel more in control. At this clear expression of core adaptive needs, the therapist promoted his sense of *agency* by directing him to say this to the catastrophizing and overcontrolling part of himself in the other chair. "Now here is where you need to say this to the other part of yourself, 'cause it's not me who's telling you to stuff your feelings, it's this other part of you. Tell this other part of yourself . . ." Once he expressed his primary needs to the other chair, the therapist directed him to switch chairs again and respond from the controlling part of himself. The goal here was to facilitate restructuring of the catastrophic cognitions. However, at this point the client was unable to continue with the exploratory process in the two chairs. He quickly became confused, agitated, and eventually said he felt completely blank. When asked to attend to his internal experience, what happened inside that made him shut down, he was simply unable to access his thoughts and feelings or to make sense of what they had been doing. The therapist *acknowledged* his anxiety and helped him accurately symbolize it, observed his shallow breathing, and suggested, "So you just made yourself very anxious, not on purpose, but somehow it automatically happened. We need to understand how you do this, so you can learn to control it." They agreed that together they needed to slow down the process and continue to explore his internal experience. They also agreed that anxiety management in the session, through attention to his breathing and bodily experience, rather than "racing" in his head, would help him control his arousal.

This illustrates exploring how maladaptive cognitions create anxiety and how in-session anxiety interfered with that exploration process. At the end of the session, the client said that he found the process very productive and explicitly stated that he did not feel judged and this increased his trust in the therapist. She responded, "I don't have a preconceived diagnosis of what's wrong and what you should do, but we explore it together, come up with some mutual understanding." This is an example of the crucial importance of collaboration in tasks and promoting client sense of control over the therapy process, in order to alleviate performance anxiety and fear of negative evaluation. In subsequent sessions, the two-chair work was used sparingly but was suggested as an option at appropriate markers. The therapist also suggested that this work was like the ultimate challenge for him, to forget the performance and attend to his internal experience, to be less externally vigilant and more internally focused. They could use his ability to engage in the chair work as a barometer of his progress in achieving his goals.

Further work entailed accessing and exploring painful childhood experiences of negative evaluation, criticism, and humiliation from his stepfather that contributed to the development of a core insecure sense of self and damaged self-esteem. This core sense of self generated his maladaptive cognitions, which in turn fueled his performance anxiety and fear of negative evaluation. Changing this self-organization then became the focus of therapy.

CHAPTER TEN

Shame

SHAME IS ABOUT feeling exposed and found lacking in dignity or worth. It involves feeling looked down upon or inferior in the eyes of others. Thus shame is closely related to fear, that is, fear of others' negative evaluation. "Shame-anxiety" makes us cautious about revealing ourselves and is at the core of a family of feelings that includes shyness, embarrassment, and disgrace. All of these feelings are characterized by self-consciousness. The development of self-consciousness, or objective awareness, may herald the innate potential to experience shame. Shame responses often develop from experiences of public failure, or being the recipient of others' scorn, contempt, and disgust. Shame then involves the experience of being looked down on by others, of contempt in the eyes of others. When the contempt and disgust of significant others is internalized and directed at the self, feelings of shame are then intrapsychically generated. This process is one of the central foci of shame-related experience in therapy.

Shame needs to be distinguished from guilt. Although they are similar, we consider shame to be a core or fundamental emotion that concerns one's worth or value as a person, whereas guilt is a more complex state that involves learned judgments about particular actions or behaviors.

The action tendencies associated with shame and guilt also are distinct. Guilt motivates atonement for wrongdoing, whereas shame is associated with the tendency to withdraw or hide. This ensures that one's flaws and personal failures are not exposed. The hiding response of shame is captured in the expression "losing face." Thus the shame response reduces facial communication (Tomkins, 1962, 1991) as the person's eyes are lowered and the upper body seems to shrink away

229

and collapse. The person can experience blushing and pounding of the heart, and awareness of oneself blushing increases the sense of looking publicly foolish or inferior. In its simplest form, the adaptive function of shame is to protect social standing and connectedness as we learn to hide that which will be judged as unacceptable. However, while shame promotes belonging and conformity to group standards, paradoxically it also produces withdrawal and isolation. The aversiveness of shame makes people hide and disavow parts of themselves and avoid situations that could invite the scorn, contempt, or disgust of others.

The emotions of contempt and disgust play a central role in generating feelings of shame, and we now will discuss the nature and function of these associated emotions. First, contempt and disgust are directed at an object that is viewed as offensive or unworthy. Disgust is a function of being too close to an indigestible object and involves a desire to expel the offensive substance. It can be thought of as an aspect of "distaste," which occurs when one tastes something disagreeable (Tomkins, 1991), but it is not limited to rejecting offensive tastes and smells. Disgust is felt in relation to anything viewed as offensive or dirty, including thoughts, values, and people. Thus some people show disgust in response to laziness, stupidity, or sexual activities and erotic ideas, for example. Contempt, on the other hand, can be thought of as an aspect of "dis-smell," which occurs in response to a foul odor (Tomkins, 1991). It entails rejection that is haughty and superior. The person raises their upper lip, pulls away their head and nose, and looks down on the other. This gives the face a look of arrogance—the perpetual critic in the presence of an offensive odor. Contempt and disgust, when directed at another for violation, serve the same adaptive function as anger, that is, they promote separation and boundary definition. However, when internalized and directed at the self, they produce maladaptive feelings of shame and self-loathing. Again, this process frequently is the focus of psychotherapy and will be elaborated on in the following discussion.

ASSESSMENT OF DIFFERENT TYPES OF SHAME

The clinical distinctions between primary adaptive and primary maladaptive shame, and between primary and secondary shame, are similar to those distinctions made in relation to anxiety. Accordingly, emotionally focused therapy (EFT) principally is concerned with not shaming clients in treatment and with changing primary maladaptive shame that is part of a core sense of self as worthless, inferior, or unlovable. Accessing primary shame for its adaptive qualities is rarely the focus of our treatment. We also are concerned with exploring and changing maladaptive secondary shame that is generated by self-critical cognitions, as well as contempt and disgust directed at the self. Secondary shame is part of a traceable sequence of feelings of unworthiness and negative thoughts that ends in a sense of self-loathing; it is distinguished from primary shame in that it is more situation specific and less chronic.

The following different types of shame need to be distinguished for the purposes of differential intervention: (1) primary maladaptive shame as a core sense of self; (2) generalized primary shame about violating values and standards; (3) secondary shame generated by self-critical cognitions and self-contempt and disgust; and (4) secondary shame about internal experience.

Primary Maladaptive Shame

There is a difference between shame as an innate emotional response to a specific situation and shame that is internalized as a core sense of oneself as worthless or unacceptably flawed. The latter internalized shame occurs through child-rearing practices that teach children that certain feelings, desires, and behaviors are unacceptable. For example, boys typically are shamed for showing weakness and girls are shamed for asserting themselves or their sexuality. Children's adaptive shame pulls them back from exposing those parts of themselves that are judged as unacceptable. Through repetition, or even an intense single experience, shame becomes internalized such that certain feelings and behaviors automatically evoke feelings of shame, whether or not the other is present. Furthermore, these shaming messages can generalize from specific feelings and behaviors to condemnation of the entire self or core aspects of the self. Views of oneself as flawed, stupid, lazy, incompetent, or selfish are based on early shaming experiences.

Shaming is a common child-rearing practice, and to a certain extent we all are damaged by it. However, the major problem is internalized shame from childhood maltreatment. People who were emotionally, physically, or sexually abused as children have internalized a sense of themselves as dirty, unlovable, or worthless. They learn to treat themselves the way they were treated by significant others, that is, with hostile self-blame and self-contempt, and this produces intense feelings of worthlessness and shame. The problem state or dysfunction is the sense that one was responsible for a shameful act over which one had no control (in the case of sexual abuse), or somehow deserved the abuse and brought it on oneself. Other forms of maltreatment can emanate from social rejection due to race, poverty, disability, or gender, and this also results in a core sense of oneself as flawed or inferior.

Obvious markers of primary maladaptive shame in therapy are chronic low self-esteem, feelings of worthlessness and inferiority, and chronic depression generated by self-denigration and self-contempt. Because a sense of oneself as worthless or defective can make people vulnerable to momentary feelings of shame, other indicators of primary maladaptive shame are intense and frequent self-consciousness, fear of negative evaluation, and embarrassment. The appropriate intervention strategy at these markers is, first, empathic affirmation of vulnerability, that is, acknowledging the pain and difficulty of these feelings. This is followed by empathic exploration of the experience, and restructuring of the emotion scheme by accessing and supporting the emergence of healthy resources.

Feelings of shame can be either acknowledged or unacknowledged. In the first instance, feelings of worthlessness and inferiority are all too painful and obvious in therapy. In the second instance, shame is unacknowledged because it is too threatening to a fragile ego or self-esteem. This commonly is observed in clients with problems of social anxiety, substance abuse, obsessiveness, perfectionism, or the grandiosity and bravado of narcissistic personality. Although these behavioral styles may protect against experiencing feelings of self-loathing and inferiority, they become maladaptive and interfere with functioning.

A person who experiences the intense humiliation and powerlessness of abuse, for example, can lash out in anger at being injured and violated. The experience of helplessness and victimization is disowned; this part of the self withdraws and cuts off in order to escape the agony of being shamed. The person fiercely defends against feelings of shame with anger and is unaware that it is the tacit underlying sense of worthlessness that is generating his or her bad feelings and maladaptive behavior. This powerful tendency to protect oneself from shame is evident in some cultural practices in which public humiliation or "losing face" was justifiable grounds for suicide or homicide to protect one's dignity or honor.

This type of secondary rage is different from the adaptive anger at maltreatment that is accessed in therapy in order to empower the individual and overcome self-blame. Maladaptive rage associated with narcissistic slights or feeling inferior, ashamed, or humiliated is recognizable because it is overly intense, chronic, or inappropriate. Intervention focuses on accessing and changing the underlying maladaptive shame. Secondary rage over a minor insult, for example, can be acknowledged by the therapist, but attention needs to be focused on how the client feels deeply wounded and can't bear even the slightest offense. This opens the door to explore pathogenic beliefs that the self is no good, or bad, so these can be exposed to new and disconfirming information. In general, whether shame is acknowledged or not, the goal of intervention is to access the maladaptive emotion scheme so that it can be modified. However, when shame is unacknowledged, the process of accessing can be more difficult.

Primary Shame from Violating Personal Standards

The distinction between shame induced by the harsh judgment of others and shame from violating one's own values and standards is an important one. The latter is observed when people feel self-contempt and disgust and is maladaptive when they cannot forgive themselves for behaviors, such as poor parenting, wasted opportunities, sexual deviation, or behavioral excesses. Here the problem is not distorted or unrealistic values and standards, or inappropriate self-blame; rather, the problem is that regrets about specific behaviors generalize to condemnation of the entire self. The action tendency becomes one of hiding the self in shame with no possibility of making amends or self-forgiveness. This inability to accept or forgive oneself can result in chronic depression, anxiety, and increased maladaptive avoidant behavior, such as substance abuse, that covers the experience of shame.

In situations in which a person is unable to forgive him- or herself for regrettable behavior or mistakes, intervention involves validating the person's values and standards and supporting their desire to "do the right thing." Affirming this desire as a healthy aspect of self supports and strengthens an alternative self-organization that counteracts condemnation of the entire self as worthless or defective.

Secondary Shame Generated by Self-Criticism

Self-criticism accompanied by self-contempt and disgust is one of the most commonly occurring dysfunctional processes associated with shame. People harshly berate, denigrate, and condemn themselves for their mistakes, flaws, or shortcomings. This generates feelings of worthlessness or inferiority, damages self-esteem, and is one of the underlying determinants of depression. The self-critical process can be activated periodically and in specific situations, or pervasively and chronically across situations. When self-criticism is pervasive and chronic it is one component of a more central (core) self-organization

and is considered symptomatic of primary maladaptive shame, discussed above.

Secondary shame can be generated by pathogenic beliefs about
oneself learned in one's culture or family of origin. Markers of this
type of shame in therapy are obvious or implied self-critical statements
accompanied by harsh vocal quality and facial expressions, such as a
curled lip or sneer that indicate feelings of contempt and disgust
toward the self. Here intervention involves highlighting or analyzing
the expressive quality of contempt, specifying the shame-producing
cognitions, heightening awareness of agency in the shame-producing
process, and countering shame by supporting the emergence of the
healthy part of self with feelings of pride.

Secondary Shame of Internal Experience

Shame often coexists with anxiety in a complex sequence of feelings
and cognitions. Secondary shame about internal experience is one
example of this relationship. Specifically, one can be ashamed of
particular emotional processes, such as feeling hurt, weak, or needy, or
feeling sexual or angry, and feeling fearful that these internal experiences will emerge. This type of shame often is similar to the avoidance
of weakness and vulnerability discussed in Chapter 9. Obvious in-
session markers are explicit negative evaluations of such experience,
or self-consciousness, or attempts to hide or avoid these experiences.
Intervention involves exploring the beliefs about experience, or empathic affirmation to help the person tolerate the shame and face the
disavowed state.

Shame-anxiety is another problem state that often is not distinguishable from feelings of vulnerability. This is anxiety about revealing
internal experience for fear of being judged, presented in the preceding
chapter. At these moments of shame-anxiety, interventions that attempt
to change or interpret the client's experience act to invalidate what the
person is feeling and counteract the innate action tendency to withdraw; rather, the best intervention is empathic attunement, support,
and affirmation of the need to protect oneself. Provision of safety and
empathic affirmation of vulnerability reduces interpersonal anxiety
and allows the person to risk revealing him- or herself. This reduces
isolation and allows the hidden aspects of self to be accessed, explored,
and exposed to new disconfirming information in the therapy session.
However, exploration of the experience takes place at a later stage,
once the intense vulnerability has passed and the client feels confident
that his or her experience is accepted.

OUR APPROACH TO INTERVENTION

Shame operates everywhere in therapy because clients are constantly concerned about what part of their inner experience can be revealed and what parts must be hidden. Therapy needs to validate clients' disclosed experiences and be careful not to shame clients by ignoring their expressions. In addition, transformation of shame about internal experiences is dependent on the empathic affirmation of another person to disconfirm pathogenic beliefs about self. Thus transformation of shame is highly dependent on the therapeutic relationship. In order to overcome shame that interferes with self-acceptance, people have to come out of hiding. However, one of the difficulties in changing shame is the difficulty in accessing the emotion scheme generating it because of the powerful tendency to hide. Emotionally focused interventions help clients acknowledge and fully experience shame, humiliation, and embarrassment, in the session, rather than avoid it, so that they can be exposed to disconfirming experiences with the therapist. Clients learn that if they reveal their flaws and shortcomings, they will not be judged as fundamentally worthless or defective. Regrettable behaviors can be acknowledged as mistakes without threatening the person's entire self-worth. Many clients report that the most helpful and healing aspect of treatment involved revealing their vulnerable, disorganized, and hidden aspects of self and having these received by another human being. The experience of simply being seen, heard, and accepted, despite one's feelings of unworthiness and desperation, is highly affirming. Clients have a new interpersonal learning and internalize the therapist's acceptance, which enhances their capacity to accept themselves.

In addition to discussing shaming experiences from the past, explorations focus on how the therapist may have shamed the client in the session by misunderstanding or missing something important. Thus immediacy in attending to how shame may be generated by the therapist's action is another important aspect of shame work. Healing these types of ruptures in the relationship and correcting current misunderstandings can be highly therapeutic and, again, provide a new interpersonal learning. In these situations, an understanding supportive relationship is not a precondition to further work with shame but is the essence of the treatment itself.

Overall, the first goal of EFT interventions to counteract shame is to develop a supportive, empathically attuned relationship. The focus then shifts to helping clients recognize and overcome avoidance in order to acknowledge painful feelings of shame. Interventions help clients bring alive and stay in touch with their experiences of shame, embarrassment, and humiliation and to symbolize these feelings in the immediacy of the session. This exposes these experiences to new information and restructures maladaptive emotion schemes. Therapy also aims at heightening experiential awareness of the process of disavowing and rejecting aspects of self, and the negative effects that this has on the individual. This awareness mobilizes healthy strengths and resources, such as compassion, self-respect, and pride, which counteract shame experiences and help to construct new meaning of shameful experiences. Mistakes or flaws can be accepted as only "part" of who the client is as a person. In these respects, working with shame is similar to working with maladaptive anxiety: treatment aims at accessing and modifying the shame structure and strengthening other essential and healthy self-organizations (Paivio & Greenberg, 1997).

Intervention Principles Relevant to Shame

Refocus Attention on Internal Experience

Deflections from the experience of shame are common because clients feel self-conscious and under scrutiny. Drawing attention to the experience can simply intensify the impulse to retreat and close down. Thus people can talk about embarrassing or humiliating experiences but avoid the intense discomfort of the immediate experience. Therapist responses such as "As you were speaking, I was aware of how degrading that must have felt" can refocus client attention on internal experience. Therapists can acknowledge the discomfort of feeling small and worthless, humiliated, dirty, especially in the presence of another, and normalize clients' desire to protect their dignity, to look away, or cover their face while they speak. Clients can be encouraged to express their reactive anger at being humiliated, but interventions should acknowledge their anger as a coping response and simultaneously should highlight the underlying core experience of shame. Here is an example of such a refocusing intervention: "Yes, so angry at him for using you. Can you get in touch with that feeling of being used? That's the important part, the damaging part. I know it's hard, it hurts, so degrading to feel ... what ... unvalued ... ?"

Sometimes it is necessary to provide a rationale in order to help clients understand the purpose of experiencing what feels like such a self-damaging emotional state. For example, when clients express reluctance to talk about embarrassing or shameful material, therapists encourage them with responses such as "I know it's hard, but it's so important to say, otherwise it eats away at you" or ". . . it keeps you so isolated." Clients with a shame-based sense of self often are highly anxious and live in constant fear of being found out and found lacking. Empathic responses can heighten awareness of how the intense impulse to retreat cuts off social contact and jeopardizes primary needs for belonging and connectedness. This accesses healthy needs and motivates clients to come out of hiding and risk disclosing shameful material.

However, directing attention to and refocusing attention on shame also can threaten a fragile ego and self-esteem. It therefore is important to assess client ego strength, to be unintrusive, delicate, and sensitive to client fragility, and to be respectful of the client's need to withdraw. It may be necessary to strengthen clients' self-esteem before they can tolerate exposing or acknowledging their experience of shame.

Present-Centeredness

As we stated earlier, people with eroded self-worth are prone to momentary experiences of shame in a variety of circumstances. They may be easily embarrassed, humiliated, and hurt, and may defend vigorously against these experiences. Therapists need to be attuned to nonverbal indicators of the emergence of shame-related experience and respond to them. These indicators include downcast eyes, squirming or writhing in the seat, and laughter or shrugging off that serves to cover embarrassment. Empathic affirmations such as "It's hard, yeah, feeling somehow foolish talking about this stuff" can open the door for further exploration. Also important are inquiries into whether the therapist has unwittingly shamed the client by not being attuned to the client's feelings or by failing to support him or her when support was needed.

Obvious and frequently occurring markers of underlying shame-related processes are explicit self-critical remarks, such as when clients call themselves "fat" or "lazy" or a "screwup." Therapist responses need to highlight the affective quality of contempt and disgust in a client's tone of voice, the arrogant tilt of the head, snarl or curl of the lip, and most importantly how it must feel to be the recipient of such contempt. For example, when a client constantly berates him- or herself for not living up to expectations, the therapist can respond, "Sometimes I get the impression that you really don't like yourself very much . . . that must be very painful to walk around like that all the time."

Interventions aimed at acknowledging shame that is on the periphery of awareness requires particular sensitivity on the part of the therapist. They involve, first, recognition of surface reactions that cover shame, such as cockiness, bravado at bad feelings, narcissistic anger, perfectionism, or other types of obsessiveness, and then, empathic conjecture about the underlying experience. These are phrased tentatively, based on knowledge of the client, and utilized only after establishment of a firm bond. An empathic response to the shame underlying a client's social anxiety is, for example, "It's almost like, if they saw you for who you really are, they'd reject you." A response to bravado about rejection might be "I hear the determination in your voice, like there's this part of you that puts on a brave front to fight against this other part that feels kind of insignificant."

For many clients, seeking psychotherapy is itself a shame-inducing experience; they feel humiliated to ask for help and admit that their life is out of control. Clients may begin a session by saying how they had to talk themselves into coming, or joke about "hating" being there, or feel "reduced to paying for help," or give any number of subtle indications that it is somehow degrading to be in therapy. Immediacy in attending to this reluctance is essential to establishing the therapeutic bond. Interventions such as "It's embarrassing to talk about such private things" or "It's hard to ask for help, feel a bit like a child" validate and open up the struggle for exploration.

Importantly, therapists also need to be attuned to spontaneously emerging challenges or adaptive resources that counteract shame. This is the part of the self that doesn't quite believe the self-criticism. For example, a client who was berating herself for "chickening out" of a direct confrontation with her parents suddenly switches to "Oh, well, at least I sent the letter." The therapist could have focused on her self-criticism or interpreted her comment as a deflection from experience. Instead, the therapist chose to support the emergence of client strength by responding, "Yes, that seems like a real accomplishment. How did it feel to put all those things on paper?" The following week, the client brought in a copy of the letter and this was used as an opportunity to explore her experience and strengthen her self-respect.

Analyze Expression

Analyzing the meaning of nonverbal behavior such as lowered eyes or flushed cheeks are important. Particularly important is vocal quality conveying self-contempt and disgust. One particularly powerful intervention consists of a two-chair enactment of the harshly negative self-evaluative processes that produce shame. At markers of self-denigration, clients are asked to enact the two parts of themselves—the critic or judge who directs contemptuous statements at the other part, the "shamefaced" recipient of all that contempt and disgust. This process heightens awareness of the specific internalized messages, the expressive quality, and the experiential impact of this contempt and disgust—the pain of such wounds and damage to self-esteem. Heightening awareness of agency in creating the experience is a crucial aspect of this intervention because it heightens clients' sense of control over their own experience.

In other situations, analysis is used to heighten awareness of the implicit messages and cognitive–affective processes that underlie and generate clients' experience of shame. Thus, in response to verbal or nonverbal markers of shame or embarrassment, clients can be asked to enact how they make themselves embarrassed, what they say to themselves to make themselves feel ashamed, in order to symbolize internalized shaming messages or beliefs about what is "wrong" with them. At times, clients will access shaming messages such as "You're so selfish" or "Homosexuality is deviant," which originate with others such as parents or society. Although therapists need to acknowledge and validate the interpersonal origins of such messages and not reinforce self-blame, eventually the client is encouraged to own the process, to view it as a belief about self that has been internalized. The shame is now internally generated, and the problem has become an intrapsychic struggle for self-acceptance. Again, this experiential awareness enhances client sense of control and agency.

Alternatively, if clients are unaware of the origins of shaming messages, exploration can focus on that. When clients are criticizing themselves, they can be asked, "Where does that come from?" or "Whose voice is that?" In either case, the purpose of the enactment or analysis is to heighten awareness of the cognitive–affective components of this intrapsychic process. Global condemnation of the self is transformed into explicit negative evaluations, and challenges to the maladaptive negative beliefs are accessed, thus restructuring the client's maladaptive shame-based sense of self.

Expression analysis also focuses on the reactions of clients as recipients of their own self-contempt and disgust. These reactions include crying, anger, or defensiveness and promises to do better. Therapist responses highlight the quality of these reactions: "feeling hostile and submissive," "feeling contrite," "feeling a little defensive," "feeling very bad about yourself," or "It hurts, like a stab or wound to yourself." Such responses foster experiential awareness of this damage to the self, and that awareness, in turn, mobilizes the healthy, self-protective part of self that will not accept such harsh treatment. Therapists support the emergence of this healthy self-structure and encourage clients to formulate an adaptive response to the shame-producing part of self. Therapists can ask clients, for example, if they can accept the harsh judgment, how they would like to respond, how they would respond if this was said to someone else; or therapists can ask clients to speak from the part of themselves that doesn't quite believe the condemnations. Thus, clients' responses of protest and defensiveness such as, "Yes, but ..." or "How dare you ..." slowly change to self-protective assertions such as "I don't deserve that" or "It's not true—I have positive qualities too."

THERAPEUTIC WORK WITH SHAME

Below we will discuss therapeutic work with the following problems related to shame: (1) generalized shame from violating personal standards and values; (2) maladaptive internalized shame generated by childhood maltreatment; (3) primary shame from social rejection; and (4) secondary shame generated by self-critical cognitions. Again, as in EFT with fear and anxiety, the emphasis is on restructuring maladaptive shame rather than on accessing primary shame for its adaptive information. Examples of core relational work are not given because this is the ongoing fabric of therapy and is occurring throughout treatment rather than in specific episodes. Examples of therapeutic work with shame of internal experience are also not presented because such work is essentially the same as working with anxiety about internal experience that was presented in Chapter 9.

Shame from Violating Personal Standards and Values

Primary adaptive shame protects social belonging; therefore, a sense of shame can result from engaging in socially and personally unacceptable behavior and violating deeply held standards and values. This type of shame is accompanied by the fear of being found out, stigmatized, and rejected, and again is similar to fear of negative evaluation. For example, in disorders such as bulimia or alcoholism that involve loss of control, or in certain types of sexual dysfunction, the client is ashamed of behavior that society may find disgusting or repugnant. He or she fears being a social outcast, and the tendency is to hide the behavior to protect his or her reputation and social standing. In other situations, the person has failed to live up to deeply held standards, for example, by being a neglectful parent or in some other way causing harm to others. The first step in treatment is to provide safety, unconditional positive regard, and matter-of-factness, in order to help the client feel safe enough to talk about the behavior. This acceptance helps to overcome shame-anxiety so that the experience can be explored. The treatment objective, in situations in which the person has done harm to self and others, is to shift overgeneralized shame and self-condemnation to regrets about the behavior or mistake and mobilize a desire to make amends. In all situations, internalizing therapist acceptance is important to achieve change.

For example, shame is a central experience for many people with a history of substance abuse. We believe that EFT is most effective once the substance abuse behavior is controlled and the person can focus on intrapsychic processes rather than behavioral change. Alternatively, EFT is carried out in conjunction with self-help programs, such as Alcoholics Anonymous, which teach important skills and provide support. Once the individual is no longer avoiding pain through substance abuse, he or she must realistically face the responsibility of violating his or her own standards and causing damage. The client often must face painful memories of degradation, loss of control, many "wasted years," loss of opportunities, loss of respect, and/or damage to self and loved ones. The pain of facing these things can lead to increased maladaptive avoidant behavior if the person cannot learn to accept and forgive him- or herself. Interventions first *acknowledge* and empathically affirm the difficulty of facing the past, and then acknowledge the client's courage in doing so. This helps to strengthen the sense of self so that when shameful material is *evoked* it can be tolerated and *explored* in therapy.

As discussed earlier, EFT interventions validate clients' regrets about specific mistakes or behaviors, their desire to feel like they belong and to make amends. These are healthy resources that can challenge and counteract a pervasive sense of oneself as a "loser" or "no good." Accessing primary unmet needs for safety, support, belonging, and acceptance also helps to motivate behavior to attain these needs. Part of the objective in unpacking the shame experience is to access and restructure a core sense of self as worthless and defective that may have contributed to avoidant and dependent behavior in the first place. Many clients who cannot forgive themselves for mistakes report, "I always felt like a loser, like I didn't fit in, that there was something wrong with me." Restructuring this core sense of self is the focus of the following case example.

Client Example

A young woman was in therapy because of relationship problems with her current boyfriend and painful resentment towards her parents. She had been repeatedly victimized by physical and sexual abuse as a girl, and exposed to extensive sexual and physical violence between her alcoholic parents. She also had been given the responsibility of caring for her younger siblings and felt hurt and angry that her parents did not appreciate her efforts and refused to acknowledge her emotional pain. In addition, she felt guilty for sometimes losing her temper and hitting her brothers and sisters and, especially, ashamed of initiating sexual experimentation with her younger brother on several occasions. She deeply loved her brothers and sisters and wanted to protect them. Furthermore, she could not forgive herself because she knew how terrible it felt to be victimized and could not understand how she could have been "abusive" herself. In her mind, she "should have known better." The therapist responded to her profound pain and regret at having hurt the ones she loves, how she wanted to be good to them: "If only you could do it all over again, you would do it differently, by the sounds of things." During one session, when she agonized about touching her brother, the therapist responded that she seemed to have the capacity to empathize with him and to imagine his pain. Further, the therapist asked, "How would you feel if you thought your parents felt the same regret and pain about hurting you?" This *evoked* the client's painful longing for recognition and acknowledgement from her parents. The client tearfully responded that she certainly could forgive them because she would then know that they cared and loved her. She was able to apply this experiential awareness to her relationship with her sibs. The week following that session, she approached her sibs, expressed her regret at the physical abuse, and asked for their forgiveness. Taking this action and their positive response helped to alleviate her guilt and strengthen her self-esteem.

However, she was most ashamed about fondling her younger brother and found this excruciatingly difficult to disclose and discuss in therapy. She hinted at it for several sessions and, finally, at the therapists encouragement—"This is eating away at you"—was able to weep and disclose what she had done. This *accessed* primary shame and beliefs about herself that she was sick, disgusting, and twisted. She hoped her brother had forgotten the incidents and was uncertain how he would respond if she "confessed." The therapist validated her inability to face her brother with the "truth" at this time, and suggested that they focus on helping her resolve the issue within herself. Then she would be in a better position to decide how to proceed with her brother.

Memory evocation was used throughout therapy to help her contact her childhood experience and get in touch with her motivation, thoughts, and feelings at the time of these troubling incidents. Again, it required considerable support, encouragement, and persistence on the part of the therapist to refocus her attention at deflections from these painful memories. The client reexperienced her anger and confusion, not knowing what she was doing but somehow copying what she had seen and experienced herself. The therapist empathically responded to her confusion, the chaos in her life, and the difficulty of a young person having to deal with these things all alone. Importantly, this exploration was done while the experiences were emotionally alive for the client; awareness emerged from the client's own experience of herself as a child rather than from an intellectual understanding of her limitations. The therapist frequently responded to her pain in talking about these incidents, highlighted her profound regret, and supported the part of her that currently knew that it was wrong and her powerful desire to do the right thing. This *mobilized* healthy resources in the form of empathy for herself, which helped to *restructure* her sense of herself as perverted and bad.

Healing and a beginning of self-forgiveness took place in an empty-chair dialogue with her brother. The therapist suggested that empty-chair work enables people to do and say things in imagination that they are not able to say in real life. This intervention could be used to help her clarify and come to terms with these issues for herself, without involving her brother. Although she experienced considerable performance anxiety, the intervention was highly evocative. The therapist directed her to say what bothered her the most about the sexual experimentation with her brother, and she expressed her fear that she had "screwed him up." Furthermore, the intervention accessed her core fear that she was sexually messed up herself and would never be able to have a normal sexual relationship. Thus core issues of sexuality were opened up for exploration. Empty-chair dialogue also *accessed* primary anger at her parents for their lack of guidance, protection, and appropriate parenting. This helped to *restructure* her self-blame and belief that she "should have known better." Other interventions included two-chair dialogues exploring self-critical processes that generated her guilt and shame. These interventions promoted her agency in producing these bad feelings and accessed challenges to these pathogenic beliefs about herself. At the end of therapy she decided not to contact her brother in real life, but she felt more resolved within herself and better able to view the incidents in perspective. She was experientially clear that her regrets and desire to make amends were genuine and that she would not do such a thing as an adult. Thus she was better able to accept herself, rather than torture and condemn herself for childhood mistakes.

Primary Shame from Childhood Maltreatment

An early learning history of rejection, ridicule, and criticism leads to deep insecurity and fear of being left alone, defenseless. These experiences can lead to the development of a core sense of self as flawed, worthless, unlovable, or bad, and therefore at risk of being abandoned. Such a core sense of self obviously is related to vulnerability, chronic anxiety, and depression.

Survivors of sexual abuse frequently feel guilty and ashamed for having transgressed moral standards and feel, somehow, responsible for the abuse. This problem state consists of inappropriately blaming the self, and consequently change involves appropriately externalizing the blame, "putting the blame where it belongs." Moreover, people who have been sexually abused feel tainted and dirty. They fear being the object of disgust and socially stigmatized, and therefore the abuse becomes a closely guarded secret. This results in pervasive shame-anxiety, hiding themselves, and fear of intimacy. Pathogenic beliefs about self were poignantly illustrated by one client who, speaking about having been sexually molested as a girl, cried, "Who would want me?" Restructuring maladaptive hiding or shame-anxiety is the objective in some treatment approaches in which abuse survivors are encouraged to "go public" about their experience. In EFT, the first step in counteracting shame involves revealing the shameful material in therapy, sharing the secret with another person who is nonrejecting and highly supportive. Anger is accessed and used as a healthy resource to externalize blame and restructure maladaptive shame by holding the abusive other accountable for harm. These are situations in which expression of contempt and disgust, directed at the abusive other, is adaptive and supported by the therapist.

Client Example

The following transcript is from therapy with a client who had been molested as a boy by his teacher (discussed earlier in Chapter 7 on anger and Chapter 8 on sadness and distress). It illustrates the use of memory evocation to access shame associated with sexual abuse, and anger to restructure his shame.

EXPLORE EXPERIENCE

T: OK, um, and you know I'm going to be aware that this is something that part of you doesn't want to deal with, you know when you tell me it's hard for you to, or you feel kinda reluctant to, and we'll just see and take it from there. (C: OK.) OK, I'm going to help you get in touch with some bodily kinds of feelings and sensations and use that as a way of getting in touch with feelings, as you remember an image um experiences from the past. You feel OK about trying that? (C: Sure.) OK, so what I'd like you to try is to maybe just close your eyes and try and make yourself as relaxed as you can, and check what's going on with you in your body, notice your breathing, any other sensations in your body, OK . . . , what you are experiencing inside, become aware of that. From time to time I'm going to ask you to tell me what's going on for you, and you can take your time to put your experience into words. Sometimes you may not have an answer, so you can just keep quiet, and just take your time to check. My suggestion is that we work with the feelings around P. [the teacher], just notice what you really feel when I mention his name, notice your breathing, can you tell me what your feeling, what's going on for you inside? [Direct attention]

C: Well, there's, huh, kinda butterflies going on (T: Mm-humm, Mm-humm.) in this area.

T: That's good that you're able to get in touch with that, sort of a nervous, jittery feeling in your stomach.

C: And, um, there's kinda of a, I don't know what you call it, closing (T: Tightness.) in the throat.

T: Uhh, OK, so stay with that experience, somehow just the mention of these experiences with P. kinda tightens. See if you can actually go back to being younger, being twelve, eleven, around the time that all these experiences were happening—what does it feel like to be S. [the client] at age twelve? [Evoke memory]

C: Huh, I remember I use to have very, physically, I used to have a very stiff style around the neck area, very stiff, very tight.

ACCESS PRIMARY EMOTION SCHEME

T: Uh-huh, uh-huh, you can remember this tightness in your neck. See if you can actually imagine or come up with some memory of being around P. when you were a kid—can you describe something, it may be fleeting images?

C: Well, embarrassment, (T: Mm-humm.) kinda mortified in front of my friends, and so I felt very small, and I remember seeing things from the perspective of being smaller than everyone else and everything else around me. Not that I was exceptionally tiny or anything as a young person, but my life felt constrained, narrow and small, um, when he entered my life. Before it used to be wide open, um, large.

T: So suddenly like he became the focus and . . .

C: Yeah, well, my whole world kinda contracted and became very small and limited, and my life used to be open and, now, there are a lot of secrets in my life, (T: Right.) um, there were constraints.

T: Stay, stay with that feeling, even if you don't keep your eyes closed, S., see if you can come up with a memory or images of being with him and maybe we can try and work with your sensory experience with him, and yourself. [Direct attention, Evoke memory]

C: Well, I have an image I can see one place in the hallway in our house.

T: Right, describe this.

C: Well, it's, uhh, the ceilings are high, there's a light hanging from a chain, there's a stairway, uhh, that winds upstairs, there's a hallway and a big front door that leads onto a very large porch, and it's a bright snowy day and I'm walking out of the door into a large open space. Uhh, he's coming over and now the room seems disproportionately, you know, constrained. Well, at the same time, I seem disproportionately small in relation to this world, and, um, everything is closed and the image of a light, is an open image, you know, I'm walking out into the open world, and now my world is closed in, and in very, very strict ways.

T: OK, just stay with this sense of feeling closed in, OK, check what it feels like to be closed, have everything so closing in on you, what does it make you feel inside? Check that feeling, S. at twelve, what is he feeling? [Direct attention]

C: Well, I'm feeling, uhh, under control, uhh, under outside control, and feeling dread, I'm feeling . . .

T: Stay with the dread, go once again into the feeling inside.

C: Well, it's the butterflies.

T: Uh-huh, uh-huh, so somehow, stay with the dread and the queasiness and the butterflies in your stomach, queasy feeling, somehow just dreading that he is coming. . . . What are you dreading about him? What he will do or . . . [Symbolize]

C: Well, I'm dreading the effect it's had, um, he created a situation which there's, we've done things, now they have to be total secrets from everyone and he's an adult, and has power and I'm a child, and I don't, and it isn't like a secret with friends of the same age, it's not that kind of secret it, um, it's the type of secret that would make, you know, that closes my life in on every side, I, I, you know, if the secret was known by my friends, by my family, um, my whole social life and my whole social world can't know about this secret, and so he has control over me now.

T: And somehow the feeling of just being alone with this secret . . .

C: Well, yeah, being alone under his control, you know it's like I'm living with my parents and I'm really under his control, and somehow my world has just collapsed around, this, um, one thing, this secret, and, uh-huh, there are many secrets and . . . I don't even want to spend time with him, I mean even aside from the sexual stuff, it's just the (T: OK.) unbalance in my life . . .

T: So say that again, say that again, and imagine him in front of you: "I don't even want to spend time with you." [Intensify]

C: No, I don't want to spend time with you, I don't want to do all these activities . . . you know, because you keep pushing that on me (*makes sweeping and dismissive gestures with his hands*).

T: Uh-huh, somehow notice what you're doing with your hands. Right, OK, as you speak you're doing this, so do this some more, put him there, and what do you say: "I don't even want to be with you"? [Analyze expression]

C: Sweeping him out of my life, dirt (*laugh*).

T: OK, so stay with that actually, and do that some more, what are your hands saying?

C: These hands are sweeping the dirt, away from me.

Access Primary Shame

T: Right, so just filth, tell more about the filth on you.

C: It makes me feel so humiliated, it is like having dirt on me, on my clothing around my body, because people can see it, they could see it, maybe they aren't seeing it, but they *could* see it, and this could be embarrassing and social, um, I could be socially ostracized, um, I don't want it on me.

T: See if there is some memory of what he did that comes up, S., uh-huh, uh-huh, just check what you're feeling inside, see if you can remember something that he did which made you feel dirty. [Memory evocation]

C: Well, I'm, I'm feeling ashamed and I don't want to say these things. . . . I don't want to say them because I'm ashamed of them.

T: Uh-huh, of course, bury them.

C: We did things that make me feel so ashamed that even as an adult I don't want to even, I can remember them, but I don't even want to say them because they're just too . . . yeah, and humiliated, they make me feel low and they make me feel, I always felt that after we did something, and I would go and relate to other people, I carried that with me, that they could somehow perceive or it didn't matter whether they could or not, that I had sex with him or did this or that, I mean I could perceive it, I mean I had just done this, right, or had done this the other day, and now I'm playing with my friends, now I'm with my parents, and now I'm here, and those memories were there, and, like I said, I just hoped he would disappear and go away all the time.

ACKNOWLEDGE AND EMPATHICALLY AFFIRM

T: Somehow powerless and just carrying this feeling . . .

C: Well, because there were these constant experiences and then I would take those experiences back with me to all the things I did and . . . um, you know, the rest of my life was, um, or could have been interesting and fun and exciting, but it was made to be, um, everything else in my life was just tainted by this, . . . I carried the memory with me, I carried the understanding and the thought with me.

T: Right, somehow the feeling inside of just being—feeling—bad and somehow dirty and having to keep this secret, to hide (C: Yeah.) is what you carried from situation to situation and that kinda colored how you felt in relating to other people. [Symbolize]

C: Yeah, well, we were doing shameful things and I felt ashamed, and I felt, you know, I felt bad! Um, I felt bad um, I felt ashamed of myself all the time and that people if they ever found out it would, but even if they didn't find out, I was ashamed of myself all the time, but at the same time I felt out of control.

T: Somehow feeling dirty but also not having control because he did this, he (C: Right.) he imposed this. [Symbolize]

ACCESS ANGER AND NEED IN ORDER TO RESTRUCTURE SHAME

T: Tell him, "You make me feel dirty," try saying that to him, so "I want you to get away." [Establish intentions]

C: Yeah, I want to, I don't know, cleanse my life of you . . . filth, worthless, garbage, junk, . . . like something dirtying everything in my life, like someone who came over and just slung mud at you all the time, and you just, um, you know his presence is just . . .

T: Uh-huh, so somehow stay with that feeling of mud being thrown at you, just something shitty being put on you, tell him how angry you are about that, him shaming you like that. [Promote agency]

C: Yeah, I am angry, you slime bag, you coerced me, you used me, sure I was curious, all adolescent boys are sexually curious, that doesn't give you the right . . .

SUPPORT AND VALIDATE

T: Yeah, you had no right to use me, take advantage . . . tell him.

C: Yeah, you absolutely had no right to do what you did.

Thus, accessing primary adaptive anger and externalizing blame helped to restructure the client's maladaptive shame. This transcript also exemplified a moment in which the client was feeling intensely vulnerable about revealing his shameful behavior and the therapist empathically affirmed his desire to hide rather than encouraging him to disclose details of the abuse. Disclosure and exploration were the focus of other sessions when the client felt less vulnerable and had more distance from his experience.

Primary Shame from Social Rejection

Sometimes a core sense of shame develops from experiences of rejection due to class, race, gender, sexuality, or being somehow "different" and judged inferior. One client, for example, felt deep shame about her infertility. This shame is not essentially different from internalized shame from childhood maltreatment, above, except that the shame is not imposed by a primary caregiver. Nevertheless, the person has internalized a core sense of him- or herself as inferior, unacceptable, deviant, or somehow deeply flawed. For example, the client with a learning disability who was mentioned in Chapter 9 on fear and anxiety had been cruelly teased in school and, through these experiences, had developed a core sense of himself as a "loser." Facing this sense of himself was excruciatingly painful. Therapy involved accessing strengths and anger at unfair treatment to help restructure this sense of himself. For people such as this man, the feelings of shame are all too present and obvious in therapy; for others, they are unacknowledged, avoided, and protected against through rage or narcissistic grandiosity and therefore need to be accessed.

The following case example illustrates EFT helping a client disclose her unacknowledged shame stemming from internalized racism.

Client Example

A black woman came to therapy because of panic attacks following the breakup of a relationship with her boyfriend. Although she acknowledged having the panic attacks, she presented herself as confident and grandiose. The therapist bypassed this surface presentation and empathically directed attention to her feelings of insecurity, her sense of impending disaster, and invited her to explore what was contributing to this. The client said that her relationship had ended because she felt ashamed of her boyfriend. She said he embarrassed her in public because of the way he dressed—"He looks like a typical lazy nigger." The therapist responded that "Somehow that rubs off on you, you're afraid that people will look down on you?" This evoked pride in how hard she worked, her drive for success, and how stressed she was from overwork. Therapist responses *validated* how important hard work and success were to her, "almost more important than anything it seems," and invited *exploration* of the meaning of these things for her. Supporting and validating the client's experience and concerns helped her feel safe and strengthened her sense of self so that she could let down her guard and reveal the more vulnerable parts of herself.

Therapist empathic responding to her intense driveness, such as "It's as if you live in constant fear that you will not get what you want, you will not succeed," *accessed* insecurity about her race and her belief that the racism of others was a barrier for her. The therapist then invited her to recall and *explore* experiences with racism: "Sure, you must have been the recipient of these attitudes many times in you life, you know what it tastes like." This *accessed* core emotion memories of her childhood, growing up as the only black family in a small town where everyone was polite, but never really feeling as though she fit in. It also accessed anger at recalled racist comments made by strangers on the street.

In situations such as this one, supporting expressions of adaptive anger at having been unfairly shamed is corrective. However, as we stated earlier, in situations where anger covers shame as core self-experience, it is more productive to help the client acknowledge the shame so that it can be restructured. Sometimes secondary anger takes the form of rage, which either can be bypassed or may need to be confronted. The most beneficial response is empathic conjecture such as "Its intolerable to feel like you do, rage against being so humiliated, being made to feel like garbage, need to protect yourself from this assault." Clients need to accept the rationale for attending to shame experience and learn to change rage into assertive expression of healthy adaptive anger at harm done to them.

In this case, the therapist acknowledged the client's anger as she recalled these abusive incidents and, at the same time, *accessed primary* shame by empathically highlighting the underlying pain of these wounds to self-esteem and pain of not belonging. Responses highlighted her longing and the adaptive need to belong: "Yeah, as kids we want so desperately to be accepted, to belong." This *evoked* tears and activated the client's core shame-related emotion scheme. She disclosed how she felt so sad and alone, as a child, wishing more than anything that she wasn't black and simultaneously feeling ashamed of that wish. The therapist validated the client's experience by responding, "Of course, as a child, being black kept you isolated and feeling somehow never good enough, so you rejected it." This helped the client feel accepted and to continue exploring her painful experience—her desperate need to be a success so she could be accepted and respected. The therapist helped her acknowledge her core feelings of inferiority, and constant struggle to prove herself, by responding, "Somehow being accepted in white society would help you accept yourself. You need this 'stamp of approval' to feel like you're OK." This helped her feel the sting of her own internalized racism, which in turn accessed challenges to the stance and mobilized healthy anger to counteract or *restructure* her internalized shame.

Therapy also explored her experience of anxiety and depression that were generated by this core sense of not being good enough. When the client remarked that she constantly fought against slipping into hopelessness, the therapist responded, "You must live with the fear that, no matter how hard you try, this will never happen, you will never be completely accepted." This *evoked* tears of hopelessness and despair, and the therapist helped her *explore* this core maladaptive emotion scheme—the sense of herself as unacceptable or inferior. Clients find this very difficult, and it requires the establishment of considerable trust and unconditional acceptance in the relationship, as well as much delicacy and attention to client vulnerability. Tentativeness in responding and references to "part" of the self that the client finds unacceptable make it easier to acknowledge. Accordingly, the therapist responded that it was difficult for the client to completely accept herself as she is—"almost as if, on some level, you don't like who you are, as if there's this part of you who believes the racist attitudes, so you're constantly struggling to hold your head up high." This promoted client agency and changed the struggle to one of enhancing self-acceptance and diminishing the need to prove herself in the eyes of others. Therapy also helped the client explore stereotypes about her race that she disliked and feared being associated with, and validated her values and standards. This *accessed* strengths and resources in the form of exploring her black culture. She was able to review her history, *renarrate* her past, and feel more proud of herself and her race.

Secondary Shame Generated by Self-Critical Cognitions

Work with secondary shame about internal experience is not essentially different from work with avoidance of emotion that was presented in the preceding chapters. The therapeutic objective is to access the underlying experience, and this is accomplished by bypassing the secondary shame or, if that is not possible, by exploring the shame-producing cognitions until a shift to more primary experience occurs. In these secondary or reactive shame responses, part of the self evaluates and feels contempt or disgust toward another part of the self. This is evident in therapy when one part of the self is the harsh critic and judge, a part that rejects certain feelings, behaviors, or characteristics of another part of the self. At the same time, the accused part of the self feels like a failure, defensive, or hostile. This cognitive–affective process is a major generating condition for insecurity, low self-esteem, and depression. Indeed, it has been argued that internally generated shame, rather than guilt, is central to depression (Kaufman, 1989).

There are numerous instances of this process. For example, failure at something the client believes one "should" be competent at entails loss of self-esteem that is generated by beliefs internalized from family or society. These beliefs are accompanied by feelings of contempt or disgust for failure to live up to the standard or to do what is required to be a good and acceptable person. The man who drinks because of a failed business or who views neediness as a kind of gross infantile deformity often has internalized such rigid standards. Similarly, women who are not successful in marriage or parenting frequently feel like personal failures. Other types of failure experiences that induce shame are poor performance in school that leaves a child feeling incompetent and stupid, shame about being depressed and seeking therapy because one "should" be able to cope, or shame about social incompetence such as not being popular or outgoing.

EFT is concerned with providing empathic affirmation of vulnerability, as well as restructuring maladaptive beliefs that underlie secondary shame, turning the contempt for the self into acceptance and self-soothing. The process of accessing and challenging beliefs differs from that used in cognitive therapy and is similar to the process described in Chapter 9 on fear and anxiety. Two-chair dialogue is frequently used to access shame-producing beliefs. This intervention highlights not only the cognitive content of the message but the contempt and disgust directed at self, along with the painful reaction of the self to this harshly negative self-evaluation. The person's awareness of agency in producing feelings of shame is heightened, and the adaptive tendency to protect the self spontaneously emerges and acts to challenge the shame messages. These are strongly supported. Clients then can begin to reevaluate and become less harsh in their judgments of themselves. They become more self-accepting and self-soothing and develop the strength to reject the negative evaluations and counteract the contempt with pride (Greenberg et al., 1993).

The following case example illustrates a single session of EFT using the two-chair intervention to explore and restructure shame associated with shyness.

Shame Secondary to Self-Critical Cognitions

This client initially sought therapy for marital distress. During the course of therapy she explored her shyness and associated maladaptive belief that something was "wrong" with her. This exploration promoted awareness of maladaptive cognitions and agency in how she stopped herself from initiating social contact. Devaluing of herself interfered with and contributed to her feeling inferior. She told herself she was uninteresting and boring. She felt inadequate, like a social failure, so she hid away, withdrew into her own world. Heightening the experience of shame generated by self-devaluation and self-disgust spontaneously mobilized her growth tendency of competence and her self-affirmation. This acted as a challenge to restructure her maladaptive beliefs about herself. The following transcript illustrates promoting ownership of negative self-evaluation attributed to others. The client begins this excerpt by saying that "others" do not accept her.

ACCESS CORE MALADAPTIVE COGNITIONS

C: I'm worried that it's something about me they don't like ... that somehow I'm not worth talking to or even acknowledging.

T: Can you change chairs. It seems there's a part of you that believes you're not worth talking to, right, makes you feel not worthwhile. We want to see how you do this to yourself, what do you say? Do this to yourself over there, make S. feel not worthwhile. [Promote agency]

C: (*switches to critical chair*) Well, I can't imagine anyone being interested in my life, it's just, I'm just not very interesting or exciting.

T: So you're not interesting, say some more. Tell this to yourself now, imagine yourself there, this is like the critical part of you. Tell her what's not interesting about her, you just ... how do you put yourself down?

C: Ok. Well, S., you don't do anything very interesting, you're boring. ... You just go to work or hang out at home. You don't do anything exciting, you don't get involved in anything, you don't make any efforts to meet people or, you just don't DO anything.

T: "DO anything," what is that tone of voice, what do you feel toward her when you say this? [Analyze expression, Direct attention]

C: I'm disgusted with her. (T: Tell her.) I'm disgusted that you don't even make an effort ... you're just so boring, you don't say anything because basically you have nothing to say.

T: Come over here, what does it feel like hearing this? [Direct attention]

C: (*switches to experiencing chair*) I think she's right, I am boring.

T: So you believe her, see this is a strong critical part of you. Come over here, do it some more about how she's boring. Tell her all the things she SHOULD do.

C: (*switches to critical chair*) You should get out more, start meeting people, you should take a course, join a club, ask people for lunch or a movie.

T: Can you come over here, what happens for you inside? [Direct attention]

C: (*switches to experiencing chair*) I think, yes, I should do that (T: But ...) but it's pointless, it's not worth the effort 'cause even if I do go out I still won't have anything to say, people will still find me boring.

T: Kind of hopeless, like it's never gonna change (C: Mm-humm.) Can you stay with that feeling and tell her what that's like for you, like no matter how hard you try you won't be able to get what you want.

C: I feel sad and depressed 'cause it's pointless, I can change what I do but it's all superficial 'cause I'm never gonna change who I am, no matter what the situation is, it's still me.

T: Like there's something fundamentally wrong with you. (C: Ya.) Come over here, so somehow there's a part of you that devalues. What's wrong with you? Depress her, how do you make her feel bad about herself, so she can't reach out. It's really important to get a feel for how you do that. [Promote agency]

C: (*switches chairs*) It's the same thing all over again, you're just not very exciting to be with, you're boring, you're not the sort of person that people want to have around (*weepy*).

T: Ya, that really hurts, say it again. [Present-centered, Intensify]

C: (*sniffles*) You're just not a person that people want to have around.

T: Ya, and that really touches the pain inside, ya? Can you come over here, tell her what that's like for you, put some words to you tears. [Direct attention, Symbolize]

RESTRUCTURE BY ACCESSING PRIMARY EXPERIENCE IN ORDER TO CHALLENGE

C: (*switches chairs*) It hurts a lot (*sniffles*) because I like to be with people, I like to joke around and do things.

T: Tell her more about that part of you.

C: Well once you get to know me, you see what's inside me.

T: Tell her what's inside.

C: There's a person that's loving, and generous, and likes to socialize, and is smart. (T: I'm smart.) I'm smart, I enjoy doing things and having fun, I'm interested in lots of things.

T: Who else would you like to say this to?

C: My husband.

T: Put him over there and tell him.

This excerpt illustrated how acknowledging hopelessness facilitates a shift to accessing internal resources that act to combat shame. We see how challenges spontaneously emerge once the client experiences the full impact of hurt and hopelessness that is produced by her own self-criticisms. The therapist then supports the emergence of these healthy resources and self-affirmations. Repeated over several sessions, this will reinforce the experience of accessing this alternate self-organization to challenge maladaptive cognitions.

Again, it requires considerable trust for clients to reveal what they consider to be their deepest flaws, what is "wrong" with them, those parts of self they are most ashamed of. Therapists need to reduce client anxiety by empathic affirmation of vulnerability and promote self-acceptance, sometimes by reframing inadequacy as insecurity. This helps to create new meaning and compassion for self.

CHAPTER ELEVEN

The Pleasant Emotions

*T*HE PLEASANT EMOTIONS play a unique, enlivening role in human experience and have been crucial in the struggle to survive and grow. They often have been overlooked or underemphasized in relation to the unpleasant or negative emotions because of the latter's more obvious and powerful impact on survival and adaptation. The pleasant emotions, particularly those emotions related to curiosity and social connectedness, however, are crucial for survival and adaptation, in that they connect the organism with the world and with others. Pleasant emotions in addition are rewarding and have motivational effects that are independent of either drive reduction or the relief of reduced negative emotion. They also enhance performance and learning. People perform better when they feel interested and happy.

Positive emotional experiences such as interest, joy, and love are therefore independent sources of motivation. They are central to mastery pleasure, to the attainment of competence, and social bonding. Interest and joy activate and guide exploratory behavior to seek out novelty and assimilate it into that which is familiar. Therefore, with their exploratory, stimulus-seeking functions, interest and joy are engines of growth and development. Similarly, by enhancing bonding, love and joy are powerful motivators of the formation and maintenance of relationships (including the therapeutic alliance).

A frequent complaint among clients seeking therapy is the absence or diminishment of interest, joy, and love in their life, leaving them feeling flat, alone, alienated, and lacking in self-confidence and self-esteem. Disorders such as anxiety and depression are characterized by stagnation and "stuckness," partly because of the lack of these emotional experiences. Intense and debilitating anxiety interferes with exploratory behavior and mastery experiences, and depression is associated with flattened affect and disconnectedness from life and relationships.

Because of the difference in the clinical relevance of pleasant and unpleasant or negative emotions, we will not provide extensive clinical examples of how to work with these. As well, therapeutic work does not provide examples of extended work, over time, with these emotions. This does not mean that they are not important nor that one does not work psychotherapeutically with these emotions. They predominantly appear as the result of change. Therapeutic work is more focused on overcoming the blocking of these emotions than on the emotions themselves. Once pleasant emotions emerge they are confirmed and elaborated, often with an aim of translating them into action. The pleasant emotions are generally blocked by other unresolved emotions or by complex interruptive process such as fear of disappointment or alienation and emptiness. Given that the pleasant emotions often are the sought-after goals of treatment, therapeutic work with them is usually brief and highly endorsing. Once interest/excitement or joy emerge they are acknowledged and sustained, and again their emergence represents a marker for helping the person move into appropriate action or contact, based on this emotion. They are expressed and enjoyed in the present, and finally when arousal has decreased they are reflected on for their significance to the person's past and future. When love or affection emerge they are symbolized and appreciated and are markers for promoting connectedness.

Clients also experience difficulty in expressing positive emotions in therapy. They may not trust such feelings as hope, happiness, or excitement. They might believe that talking about them will change them or make them disappear. Most importantly they might fear that the therapist will not pay these experiences the attention they deserve and in not doing so will invalidate them. Recognition and support of their emergence is thus crucial to confirm and strengthen the growing positive emotions, signifying that these experiences are relevant and important. Some clients wonder if their positive experiences belong in therapy; some wonder if their therapist expects them to forever feel positive; or some worry about letting down their therapists if their positive feelings are not maintained. Therapists need to reassure their clients that their positive emotions are as important and fluid as bad feelings.

One of the major sources of pleasant emotion in therapy is the therapeutic relationship itself, where clients feel both the joy of being understood and respected, the interest and caring of their therapists, as well as feeling their own interest in reciprocal caring for the therapist. Without these positive emotions there would not be a strong enough bond to sustain a good working alliance. A rupture in the positive emotional connection between client and therapist will produce shame, fear, anger, and sadness in the relationship itself and this will impede further therapeutic work unless attended to. Thus the pleasant emotions are highly significant in the relationship and act as a kind of barometer of the therapeutic alliance. Therapy needs constantly to support and nurture the development of these emotions.

In this chapter, we first will review the emotions of interest/excitement and happiness/joy. Interest is not thought of as an emotion but rather as an index of arousal associated with a variety of emotional states. We will argue, however, that interest is one of the most fundamental emotions, that it is highly prevalent in human experience, and necessary in proactive adaptation. It is also important to note that there is a strong reciprocal relationship between excitement and joy in that a person can enjoy excitement and be excited by enjoyment. The interrelatedness of these two emotions is so prevalent that we will treat them together in discussing their effects on curiosity and connectedness.

INTEREST/EXCITEMENT

Interest is the most frequently experienced positive emotion. It is an important motivator of many actions and is important in guiding perception and attention. Interest is present in ordinary consciousness at most times and change or novelty are the key determinants of interest.

Interest/excitement involves both arousal and orientation, and the response is both passive and active. In the first type a person can be passively fascinated by an object. *Inter-est* means to be among or to "dwell in" something. It is an experience in which attention is fully absorbed: the person is breathless and the gaze is full. In the other type of response a person is excited about something, rapidly exploring the object, breathing rapidly, and actively trying to maximize information about that object. Excitement thus can be sufficiently intense to motivate motor action and amplify sexual stimulation, as well as being sufficiently graded to support subtle cognitive activity and maintain long-term effort and commitment.

In our view both interest and excitement are primary sources of human motivation. Excitement is not a derivative of drives, but a major source of motivation acting to intensify efforts at goal attainment. Interest is the primary force that keeps people actively engaged in contacting the world. Curiosity linked to the cognitive and perceptual systems sustains the analysis of the environment independent of drives such as hunger and thirst. Without interest one no longer engages with the world, no longer explores possibilities or is curious about novelty. To have no interest would be equivalent to being dormant—lacking in sensory input and without cognitive stimulation. The absence of interest seriously impairs sensorimotor, perceptual, and cognitive development, and this is manifested in depressive states. In fact, interest in combination with excitement/joy supports the operation and development of motor and perceptual processes as well as cognitive assimilation and other processes involved in cognitive development and learning. In order to voluntarily do something and to engage in much activity, one must be excited, one must be interested. Natural curiosity in regard to novelty is thus a key motivator of life; it is what keeps people going. Again, as in depression, its reduction or loss leaves people listless and impaired.

Without the capacity to continuously explore and process novel information, one is less adaptively organized for dealing with dangers and new possibilities. Thus the impaired capacity for exploratory behavior associated with chronic anxiety, for example, contributes to dysfunction. Knowing about their environment equips people to deal with it most effectively. Thus interest supports both survival and growth. Interest in goal attainment is also crucial in sustaining achievement, while the quest for new experience driven by interest and curiosity is the source of creativity.

Interest and excitement also are central in sexual experience and striving. Without these emotions sex would be dull and boring and not as motivationally charged. These emotions are therefore evolutionarily crucial not only in keeping people active in making contact with the world but also in keeping them active in pursuit of sexual experience.

HAPPINESS/JOY

Happiness and joy are distinguishable from excitement and interest both in response pattern and experienced quality. While interest is associated with attention and learning, happiness is associated with laughing and smiling and is experienced as highly pleasurable. Some animals such as cats and some monkeys emit a joy sound of purring. Happiness is one of the most desirable of states for all of us and often refers to a broad state that applies to life as a whole—to the attainment of that which is most profoundly desired and global, that all is right with us and the world.

Enjoyment arises from diverse causes. The smiling response is activated early in life by the face of the caretaker, by the sudden appearance of something familiar, by the appearance of distortions in the familiar, and by the achievement of the sought-for results of one's own efforts, that is, "getting it right." The smiling response and the experience of joy in response to the human face are both highly rewarding. Joy thus complements interest and sadness in guaranteeing that we will be social creatures. The experience of excitement at goal attainment also leads to joy in relation to the inanimate environment. It feels good to be effective, and this keeps us engaged in projects. Play is another area in which we feel the adaptive organizing effects of positive emotions. Joy is achieved by the repetition of behaviors that provide mastery and the attainment of a shared goal with another person, for example, in games.

The evolutionary significance of social responsiveness and therefore of joy is apparent. Expressing pleasure in actively engaging others has adaptive significance. It attracts the care of the caretaker and enhances mutual responsiveness because both the infant and the caretaker are continually rewarded by each other's presence. Thus it is easy to see how the absence of joy and emotional flatness associated with adult depression can interfere with responsiveness from others, disrupt emotional bonds, and exacerbate the depression. Smiling in response to the human face is the root of much human connectedness independent of feeding and touching. In infants, smiling facilitates bonding in the loving relationship, adds feelings of warmth and pleasure, and provides the caregiver with feedback about what is pleasing to the child. Among adults, smiling has the capacity to operate as a universally recognizable signal of readiness for friendly interaction. In addition to the positive role of smiling in bonding, the sharing of positive affect, positive emotional communication, and caregiver affirmations, all provide crucial encouragement for growth and development of the self. Emotional availability of the caretaker is essential in facilitating development. Interchange of interest and enjoyment, and excitement and joy, between the infant and the caregiver is a sign of healthy development.

Presence of a sense of humor in a client seeking therapy is one prognostic marker for the capacity to develop a therapeutic relationship and to change. In addition, the therapist as caregiver in emotionally focused therapy (EFT) is not "neutral" but is highly empathically attuned and responsive to positive as well as negative (painful) affects. Therapists share and support clients' positive emotional experiences. Interventions respond to, direct attention to, and facilitate exploration of emotions of interest, excitement, and joy, focusing on their growth-enhancing potential. These experiences are acknowledged in order to heighten awareness, clarify values, strengthen the sense of self, and promote healthy development. Often, positive emotion is buried in what we have called the client's "hidden essential self." Interventions direct attention to positive emotions as they emerge or access them through memory evocation.

Action Tendencies

The action tendencies of the positive emotions are less clearly differentiated from each other than they are in the negative emotions. Whereas negative emotion is associated with tension and physiological closing down, positive emotion opens us up physiologically and tension is released. We look at others (or objects) with a full gaze, or the eyebrows are down and we track, look at, and listen to what's happening with interest. Both interest and excitement involve opening the individual up to information. Thus, in therapy, relaxation exercises and attention to bodily tensing are designed to allow release of tension and to open the individual up to information and positive emotional experience.

Similarly, the experience of happiness/joy involves expansiveness. Laughter is a more primitive form of enjoyment, which later becomes differentiated into advanced responses like the smile, the chuckle, the giggle, the guffaw, and the belly laugh. Laughter thus is a complex and energizing response that involves breathing, facial muscles, and the entire body. For example, people describe doubling over from laughter, or laughing so hard their stomach hurts. Much has been written recently about the health-promoting qualities of laughter.

Problems

Most problems related to positive emotion have to do with their diminished presence or their total absence and it is these types of problems that we concentrate on in EFT. However, pathologies of excess in this domain may relate to mania and addiction (Tomkins, 1962). In mania, the person is too excited and insomnia may result. There is too much excitement that is undifferentiated (i.e., not selectively reactive to circumstances). In addiction, the person becomes attracted to some substance that produces intensely rewarding gratification with attendant blissfulness and euphoric excitement. The person then becomes dependent on or compulsively and habitually uses the substance to reproduce the joy/blissful gratification and euphoria. Although there is controversy about the definition and nature of addiction, one conceptualization is that in any experience in which the presence of an object is intensely rewarding or self-gratifying and the absence is highly punishing, there is the potential for a form of addiction. Joy, then, in a similar way, is one of a complex of emotions that can be organized so as to promote the formation of psychological addiction. The experience of joy also can be sufficiently rewarding to enable people to overcome fear, shame, and distress, and the reduction of these negative feelings can promote dependency on whatever produces the feeling of joy.

The problems we deal with most frequently in EFT are, of course, related to the absence of joy, as in depression, as well as inhibited exploratory behavior and mastery experiences in both anxiety and depression. As well, we frequently encounter pathology involving absence of positive emotion in the emotional numbing associated with traumatic experiences and posttraumatic stress symptomatology. The defensive shutting down of painful memories and experience, as a strategy for coping with overwhelming intrusion of these experiences, can generalize to numbing of all emotional experience. Clients report that their overall capacity for emotion is diminished.

General Therapeutic Perspective

Clearly, the process of accessing the positive emotions of interest/excitement and joy is different in many ways from accessing the more painful or problematic feelings. However, the goal, as with other primary adaptive emotions, is to attend to and access these emotions in order to inform action. In the early stages of therapy, where absence of positive emotion is a problem, attending to this absence can evoke a kind of longing for this lost part of self. Interventions that direct attention to and heighten this longing enhance motivation to access this hidden essential self.

Interest/excitement and joy, however, often arise as the result of a therapeutic change process, rather than as a part of it. They are an end point of a change process. In the following example we see the client's interest/excitement emerge; she uses the metaphor of a growing seed to capture this emergence of interest in life and excitement about possibilities:

T: So somehow this process has helped you to feel more . . . like you know . . . [Symbolize]

C: This is me.

T: What you are.

C: What I am. And if I decide to go that route, it's OK. If I make a mistake, then its only my fault and nobody else's.

T: And I guess that's pretty important because it's a starting place in a way.

C: Yeah, it feels like this planted a seed, and no one can take that away form you. Like you say, its a starting point of planting that seed, and going back to it, and just being more involved interested and a little more understanding here, or . . .

T: So somehow it helps you in the world, right? I mean, you have, you can always work from that place. And sometimes life is difficult, or sometimes things are sad or lonely and hard, and yet you have an ability to go back and feel that. [Establish intentions]

C: Yeah, and that part is an accomplishment to me. I feel strong and pleased about it. More alive, excited.

T: Yeah. That's important, that's nice for me to hear.

C: Yeah, as me coming here, and what I've accomplished. I think its a lot . . . in a short time. It's not years and years.

Another client in the final session talks about his happiness with his progress in treatment:

C: I am tremendously happy with the strides that we have made. Coming out the end of this process, I would have to say, I'm almost a new person. You know, there are things that I have to work on, but I've made some tremendous tremendous strides. I don't know me, to a great extent (*laughs*). So in that way, yes, I am very very happy. I am no longer, the depression is gone. It's just not a thing any more. Remember I was talking about death originally. Well, right now I could understand how I could have gotten to that stage. A person is so deep and depressed that they don't have a clear perspective of what everything is all about. I've come a long way, a hell of a long way. I think I'm gonna enjoy it, OK, getting to where I have to go from here. So it's been absolutely, it's been an experience of a lifetime for me.

The following excerpt shows a dialogue between two sides of the person in which excitement/interest is not the result of treatment but part of integrating a previously opposing aspect of self. In this excerpt a more social side of the client has been disavowing a dark and creative side which is beginning to emerge:

C: I feel that I'm awakening and starting to stretch my muscles, a potential for coming out. I'm starting to feel more confident that I am going to come out and that I will be accepted and be useful.

T: What does the other side say, the light social side? [Symbolize]

C: The light social side from this side of me, I'm quite excited about that. I see that the door is ajar. I see that the tendrils are starting to come out of the other side, and I know that the possibility is now there for joining the two, but I don't feel any pressure right now to reach into the other side. I feel that the time will come when I will do that. I know that once I'm at our cottage in July there will be more opportunity for that.

T: Will you come over here [chair]? Make contact. Speak to her. Tell her. [Promote agency]

C: Most of the time, I'm not scared of her.

T: See if you can actually make contact. What do you see?

C: I think there is something quite interesting there I'm interested to meet.

T: Tell her, "I'm interested to meet you."

C: "I'm looking forward to meeting you on equal ground somewhere. I don't feel that my life right now is on equal ground. I feel that I am much more on this social side of me than I have to be right now, but I'm looking forward to meeting you away from here on mutual ground."

Once interest/excitement or joy have been activated in the course of treatment they are worked with according to the general principles of intervention. For example, in the following excerpt, where a momentary good feeling is attended to, it is focused on and intensified in a present-centered manner.

C: I just feel it inside. I'm not afraid of it anymore. I'm not afraid to show that I am, that I have weaknesses. I am a little, don't get me wrong—I am a little. You know, I am not going to all of sudden go off and let the whole thing down, but yeah, I . . .

T: Do you still have to show your family that you're strong?

C: Well, put it this way: There is a strength in just doing. Whether what you're showing is a weakness, that in itself is a strength, OK, but that comes from within. That doesn't come from without. That felt good for a second! To tell you the truth (*laughs*).

T: Can you expand that so we don't lose it? What felt good? [Direct attention, Symbolize]

C: That felt good that I really accepted that there is a strength in showing a weakness. That's something that you don't need anyone else outside you to see—that, that's just a good feeling that comes from inside. That, I don't know, it's hard to explain.

T: There's a strength in accepting who you are, without the pushing.

C: Without any pushing, yeah. That's the strength, yeah. [Symbolize]

T: That's where the strength comes.

C: And that's really where the strength should be.

In the following excerpt from another depressed client a feeling of excitement is affirmed and supported.

C: For argument's sake, let's take Wednesday. Just going in there completely open and free. If it collapses, it collapses. That's what happens. If it doesn't, let's see what happens.

T: So are you saying, "I'm willing to go along with this experiment"?

C: Yeah. Let's see what happens. Let's just let her go. Wow! That's close to me saying what I've been saying. I need to come out, to go downtown and just pick a spot on a main street, and just go yelling and screaming, up and down the sidewalk. Just do it, just do it!

T: (*laughing*) What would you be yelling and screaming? [Symbolize]

C: Just do it. Just for the sake of letting everything go. Just throwing all caution to the wind. And not being concerned anywhere beyond that. This is close to it.

T: What's the feeling?

C: Actually, it feels good, it is starting to feel pretty good. Just, I think that is the way I need to go. I think this feeling that I'm having here, for an instant there, and for a little bit, I started to feel like a little bit of a good feeling, and not a pressure feeling. Not able to build on it, its just there, but . . .

T: It's the beginning of something.

C: Yeah.

T: Just throw all caution to the wind, my God.

In further applying intervention principles, memories of happy moments can be evoked and the person can be encouraged to own their capacities for positive interest, excitement, and joy. For example, in Chapter 9 on fear and anxiety we discussed a client's development of an insecure self from growing up in a violent home. The client's lifelong timidity was debilitating in terms of her accomplishing things and feeling self-confident. At one point the client recalled a time of feeling free and unburdened. The therapist helped her explore this memory, attend to her internal experience at the time, the lightheartedness, the confidence, the freedom, the strength and openness in her body. When tears welled up, the therapist responded to her pain and sadness at the loss of this part of her self and her longing to reconnect with that self. This was a powerful experience of her desired goals for therapy and life. The "hidden essential self" is an extremely useful metaphor that clients can relate to, and time is spent exploring how this essential self went into hiding.

Another client realized that all her life she had been waiting for her fear to go away so that she could get on with her life. Her fear had been debilitating and prevented her from doing and trying all kinds of things in her life. Interventions directed attention to this experiential burden, to "the shackles and the frightened little animal inside." Therapy focused on helping her feel and acknowledge her fear and to gradually try things in spite of her fear, "do it anyway." She began to try new things and shared her accomplishments in therapy. The therapist supported these accomplishments, shared her joy and experience of mastery and her increased confidence. Interventions directed attention to those good feelings, helped her symbolize the experience she felt in her body, and explicate their meaning to her life. Successes built more confidence, and she reveled in this new experience of mastery. The mastery experience itself was motivating. One important area for this client was fear of her own feelings and avoiding painful internal experience, which also contributed to her alienation and disorientation. She was able to apply her new confidence to allowing and accepting previously threatening aspects of her own experience. Thus, she was able to let go of some control and, again, relax and open up to new experience and information. The therapist continually helped her to articulate her excitement at self-discovery.

One feature of the present-centeredness principle in EFT can be observed when clients cancel out or deflect from painful experience by commenting on the positive side. This need to balance the scales is not only viewed as a deflection from experience but also is acknowledged in its own right. Interventions acknowledge polarities in client experience. For example, a depressed client came to a session feeling quite hopeless, but rather than exploring her struggles she reported all her successes in managing her depression and anxiety. The therapist, rather than refocus her on her evident current painful experience or confront her deflection from this experience, acknowledged her success and encouraged exploration of her struggles. Interventions that highlighted her strengths allowed her to explore her struggles and contributed to developing a stronger sense of herself.

Another example is of a client who was depressed and felt stuck in an unhappy marriage, living a flat and joyless life. An important part of therapy was helping her attend to and explore her memory of a time when she was having an affair—how alive she felt, how much she wanted and needed to feel loved, and the effect this had had on her life, providing confidence, and a sense of well-being. Accessing these positive emotions and her healthy needs and desires helped motivate her to find ways to seek them out in her marriage as well as to overcome her fear of leaving if she could not find them in her marriage. When clients report shifts to suddenly experiencing more positive emotion, it is important to explore this. For example, a depressed client whose presenting complaint was that she felt no joy and could not seem to appreciate her life suddenly began to experience more moments of joy. It was important to evoke a situation in which this occurred and then to help her attend to her internal reaction to the situation and to reexperience and explore how the change came about. This helped her become aware that feeling liked by others evoked her more positive mood and this was empowering. She thereby experienced some understanding and control over her experience, rather than believing that these moods magically descended and could magically disappear as well.

Finally the creation of hope is of crucial importance. Although hope is a complex emotion beyond the scope of this book, it is related to joy and excitement. A book on emotion in psychotherapy would be incomplete without commenting about hope, because it is such a central ingredient in overcoming discouragement and producing change. An excerpt on hope is therefore included:

C: But I'm glad the depression is gone. That part makes me feel hopeful.

T: Uh-huh hopeful.

C: Hopeful, mmh. For myself, more than just overcoming . . . um . . .

T: For yourself . . . ?

C: I'm more sure. I'm more sure of myself. That's what I'm trying to say. Making certain decisions now isn't so confusing. It's . . . there's more of a clear picture.

T: Hhm, like you have more clarity to make decisions. [Symbolize]

C: I like to stick through them, which before I found that I could be talked out of them much easier than now. Now I'm more firm.

T: You're more firm, mmh. It's nice to know what you want.

C: And the assurance. I guess . . . I assure myself that I'm OK . . . "I deserve that" or "I'm worth it."

T: Hmm, so you can kind of give yourself a positive stroke when you need to. It's OK for you to stand up for yourself. [Establish intentions]

C: Yeah. I just . . .hang in there and don't give up.

Thus, positive states are symbolized and the direction for action, goals, and intentions that they embody are articulated. Establishing intentions and setting goals in these states is important, for this sets up a positive view of possibilities and a sense of what to aim toward. Detailed planning of how to implement these goals should not be emphasized while people are in an expansive state. This should be done later, but a clear general vision or goal should be symbolized along with deep experience of "how good it feels."

LOVE/AFFECTION/CARING

Love is fundamental to human nature. It appears universally in some form, and appears to be a part of our biological heritage. There are a number of ways in which love differs from the other discrete emotions. Although love appears to be basic and fundamental, it differs from sadness or joy, which have identifiable expressions, more specific feeling states, and patterns of action. Love is more complex than the other basic emotions and may involve patterns of emotions, cognitions, and drives. There is thus no single definition of love, probably because there are several types of love, each with different types of connotations. A distinction, for example, is readily made between romantic or passionate love and compassionate or platonic love. Then, there is mother love, father love, sibling love, or friendship—all are different.

Love in the most general sense is an emotion that connects us to others and is our response to what we value most highly. It may be a derivative of other emotions, especially of joy and excitement. Love is to a large degree the experience of joyous excitement in interaction or involvement with another. It is, however, a special type of joy. It involves taking delight in the person whom one loves and finding fulfillment and pleasure in being in contact with the other. Love seems to involve an expansion of the self. In making contact with another we ourselves become, not only more whole and more integrated, but also expanded, incorporating aspects of the other into the self, developing new skills, attitudes, and resources and a greater ability to survive and grow. We experience the loved one as a source of fulfillment for important psychological needs.

Love commonly refers to a complex relationship rather than a momentary emotional state. However, love, as a discrete emotion, does refer to a momentary state, a feeling of affection that comes and goes. When people feel loved they experience momentary states of bliss and joy, they generally feel accepted and understood, and experience a sense of union; they also feel safe and secure and more self-confident. Passionate love, as well as being filled with excitement and longing, is also fraught with anxiety, despair, loneliness, and intense fear. Passionate love involves an intense longing for connection or union with the loved person and often results in joy and fulfillment. Companionate love is far less intense than passionate love but involves commitment and intimacy.

The need for adult intimacy appears universal, and intimate relationships are important sources of social support that enhance well-being and protect people from stress and ill health. Love can be viewed as a form of adult attachment rooted in childhood experiences of attachment; therefore, it is subject to some of the same processes that occur in childhood attachment, including anxiety about separation and loss. The experience of an attachment bond then appears to be a fundamental human and primate experience, and the desire for intimacy and connectedness is an aspect of mature human interdependence. In a secure adult attachment bond, people are mutually emotionally accessible and responsive.

Attachment in infants is crucial to survival. Although the emotions of anger and fear associated with fight or flight are crucial to survival, the infant comes into the world with the capacities to clutch and cling, which are the first capacities for survival. The earliest stage of a child's life is dominated by dependence and helplessness in which the child is totally reliant on the caretaker. Love is the means by which helplessness is transformed into security. The danger lies in feeling helpless and unloved, and it is this threat that is the source of separation anxiety. The loving and caring capacity appears to be innate, although complex, and is somewhat dependent on having received love and care oneself. People do, however, appear to be naturally caring, responding to the small, the childlike, and the helpless with care.

It appears that feeling cared for by another helps alleviate anxiety. From the earliest stages of development through adulthood and old age, care and empathy helps individuals regulate their own affective states and their anxieties. A sense of confidence or competence comes from appropriate empathic attunement by the other. For infants, being cared for by caretakers provides the basis for the development of a secure self. Caring does not just occur in the parent–child relationship. Rather, it is part of the relationship between peers and flows from child to parent and between therapist and client. Being connected—in emotional contact—appears central to well-being. Separation, loss of contact, and isolation are one of the most dreaded of human states, a fate comparable to death. The threat of the withdrawal or loss of another's love is terrifying to many, and this threat is at the root of a core insecure sense of self and anxiety disorders. Moreover, a common complaint among clients seeking therapy is the fear that they are themselves cold and incapable of deep caring and love. This is often a part of the flattened affect of lingering depression or schizoid-type personality problems characterized by chronic interpersonal alienation and isolation.

Action Tendency

The emotion of love entails the action tendency to make some form of contact with the loved one and a disposition to evaluate the other positively and as profoundly important for one's well-being. In romantic love the tendency is an urge for intimacy and physical affection from the loved one, including concern, warmth, tenderness, and sexual contact. There is a strong desire to touch and be touched. This is also the case in parent–child relationships, and clients often feel profoundly sad and doubt that their parents loved them when they have been deprived of physical contact and hugs. It is a common complaint that "He never hugged me" or "She never liked to cuddle me." It seems it is difficult to truly feel loved without this. In platonic love or liking there is a desire for social and personal intimacy, and although it is nonsexual it still involves interest, warmth, and concern for the other. Again, caring is powerfully communicated through physical contact and highlights the potency of therapeutic touch, which will be discussed in Chapter 12.

Researchers have attempted, with some success, to pinpoint facial expressions involved with love and have found that people may be able to distinguish facial expressions of love from that of other primary emotions (Ekman & Davidson, 1994). Exactly how people do this is not yet clear, but it may be that the face takes on the look of mothers happily, tenderly gazing at their infants. In the context of therapy, clients easily recognize tenderness, unconditional positive regard, and the genuine caring of their therapists.

Problems

Problems that arise from this emotion are a dependence on others, to the point where the person feels unable to survive without the other, or problems of one-sided or unrequited love. The reciprocal problem is an impaired capacity for experiencing the love of another, as in coldness and extreme self-centeredness. Attachment disorders, basic insecurity, and separation anxieties are also related problems. The clinging and rage associated with anxious attachment, and the isolation, aloofness, and pathological independence associated with avoidant patterns of attachment, are all related to difficulties with love, intimacy, and caring. The fear of intimacy is a central relationship problem experienced by many in and outside of close relationships.

Phobias, especially agoraphobia, can involve basic insecurity and fears of separation. In agoraphobia, for example, the terror is separation from home. People who feel unable to cope recall times of feeling safe and loved at home often in early childhood and seek out similar situations. Dependent and anxious people often are more likely to fall passionately in love. Anything that makes adults feels helpless and dependent as they were as children, anything that makes them fear separation and loss, tends to increase a passionate desire to merge with someone. However, accessing memories of early childhood safety and love also can serve as coping tools. One highly anxious client reviewed a family album in therapy and discovered photographs of her father holding her when she was a little girl. Up to this point she could only remember family violence and feeling afraid as a child. She was uncertain whether her father had ever held her. This photo became a symbol for her and proof that she was loved by him. She described the discovery of this photo as a turning point in which she began to feel more "centered" and in control.

Love, then, which is sometimes joyously exciting, also can result in a great deal of pain, misery, jealousy, uncertainty, anxiety, and despair when not received, and can result in dependence-related problems.

General Therapeutic Perspective

Again, the process of accessing love in individual therapy differs from the process of accessing the negative emotions. The goal, however, is similarly to access the adaptive striving associated with the primary emotion. The experience of love will motivate contact and caring actions. This is illustrated by a client who in anger had cut herself off from her adopted son. This was resolved in an empty-chair dialogue in therapy in which facing him in imagination accessed her love for him. This, in turn, accessed intentions to contact him and maintain contact. Accessing love for the other is commonly a part of resolving interpersonal issues in therapy, such as unfinished business with a parent or spouse.

Love is evoked in order to access the positive affiliative tendencies toward others and for the intrinsic meaning that this emotion gives to life. It is helpful to symbolize love-expressing and -evoking words because they are often taken for granted or overlooked, though they are among the prime motivating forces in making intimate relationships work. It is significant that clients feel embarrassed to express love or are frightened of the intensity of their feelings. Also, clients fear expressing love for another for fear of being devastated if their love is not reciprocated. These are blocks to the expression of love that need to be worked through in therapy in order to access the healthy motivating aspects and meanings.

Thus, problem states in therapy related to love generally result from other unresolved emotional issues that prevent love from being experienced. Feelings of alienation, deadness, or inability to love usually result from other complex processes, and accessing love is a result of resolving these other issues rather than being worked on directly. Accessing love in interpersonal relationships is a key goal of therapy and a central capacity of healthy functioning. In our therapeutic work, love often emerges in empty-chair dialogue with a significant other and generally represents an aspect of the resolution of unfinished business. This is demonstrated in the following excerpt:

T: It also feels like today, in what you were saying to your parents, there are very strong feelings, and many different strands of feeling. It's not just one monocolor, kind of thing.

C: No, it isn't.

T: You know, there was resentment, and anger, and disappointment. There's also love. [Direct attention]

C: There's a lot of love. I feel compassion, right now, for my parents. When you come out the other end of a process, you do, you feel compassion for them.

T: Would you like to sort of finish off . . . ?

C: (*speaking to the empty chair*) I love you two very very much. I really do. I need your help, to get through this process. Let's, for the first time in our lives, at least for me, anyway, even if its not for you, let's really feel a love feeling together, and cherish that what we have, more than anything else. We can't—in fact, if you look at it, we can't do without it. We couldn't come out the other end not wanting and loving one another. Once we show each other who we are as people, I think we're going to love one another very very much. Its never too late for that. I love you, even considering all that's happened, and all that has been done. I not only love you, I need you. Stay with me, and help me. You know, if I talk to them personally that way, they'll be there. They'll express their love. They don't know completely what it is that we are. We like to think that they know a little of where we are, but they don't, and they really can't completely.

T: Are you saying you have to show them? [Establish intentions]

C: Yeah, they have to be. It's one thing for me to sit back and criticize them for not approaching, but I'm a full adult now, so I can no longer throw it to that side. I have to now come out, and help them to help me. (T: Yes.) And it becomes a reciprocating process. And it will, there's no question. I mean the love in our family, boy, its strong. I mean you can't have nine kids in a family—maybe an inherent part of that, that process—but you can't have nine kids that grew up in a three-room house, that shared everything, you know, that depended and relied on one another . . . That growth, and that feeling, that part of you, no, it doesn't go away. That's a reason for being.

An excellent example of the powerful role of accessing love and caring was given in Chapter 9 in the discussion of therapy with a client whose mother had committed suicide. Memory evocation techniques accessed experiential memories of her mother's nurturing and caring, memories that had not been available to her for 35 years. These experiential memories helped restructure her maladaptive beliefs about her mother and their relationship. This, in turn, helped her feel unconflicted love toward her dead mother and feel warmed and healed by this experience. Another common example of accessing love and caring in therapy concerns accessing self-care and self-soothing for clients with a core insecure sense of self and who have difficulties with self-soothing. Again, memory evocation strategies can help clients experience themselves as little frightened children and help them to soothe and comfort themselves. These experiences can have a powerful and highly evocative impact. Clients who otherwise are unable to access tender feelings often respond with caring and tears to images of children.

Another area where accessing love is important is in situations where clients cannot seem to reconcile the conflict between love and hate or intense anger toward a loved one. This is common among clients who have been abused as children. Sometimes it is important to access the love and acknowledge and express this before clients can feel comfortable expressing their intense anger. For other clients, fully experiencing and assertively expressing anger can access love. Interventions need to highlight both sides of the conflictual experience. By attending to and experiencing both, clients learn that sometimes both experiences are legitimate aspects of mature, intense interpersonal relationships. Several examples have been given in earlier chapters, and we will not provide further examples here.

Although we have treated the pleasant emotions in a far briefer manner than the unpleasant ones, we do not wish to underemphasize their importance in life and as a goal of treatment. When people feel these feelings they predominantly do not require therapeutic intervention, however, and this accounts for the briefer coverage. What blocks the natural emergence of excitement, interest, joy, love, and caring has been the major focus of the chapters on working with the negative emotions.

CHAPTER TWELVE

Research, Training, and Supervision

W E HAVE PRESENTED the general theory, intervention framework, and intervention principles of emotionally focused therapy (EFT) and applied these to therapeutic work with specific emotions. We will conclude with a brief review of research and a discussion of clinical training and supervision. Our approach to training and supervision grows out of theory and research that has a high degree of specificity. The theory defines not only general models of functioning and dysfunction but also provides empirically based models of particular affective tasks, dysfunctional processes, and mechanisms of change (Greenberg et al., 1993).

RESEARCH

Empirical support for the efficacy of an emotionally focused approach has been generated for populations with major depressive disorder and for clients who have suffered childhood maltreatment or have unresolved interpersonal problems with significant others (Bergin & Garfield, 1994; Paivio et al., 1996; Paivio & Greenberg, 1995; Greenberg & Watson, in press). Related process research on these populations has explicitly defined types of interventions, in-session processes, and mechanisms of change related to outcome (Goldman, 1995; Greenberg, 1979, 1984, 1994; Greenberg & Foerster, 1995; Greenberg & Hirscheimer, 1994; Watson & Greenberg, in press). This type of detailed process research helps conceptualize the process of therapy in very specific terms. Extensive research has also demonstrated the effectiveness of an emotionally focused approach with couples and studied the process of change (Goldman & Greenberg, 1992; Gordon Walker, Johnson, Manion, & Cloutier, 1996; Greenberg, Ford, Alden, & Johnson, 1992; Johnson & Greenberg, 1985, 1988).

TRAINING

Training in EFT focuses on developing conceptual, perceptual, and intervention skills. In this approach developing an understanding of theory and abstract concepts is enhanced by experiential awareness of the concepts. Thus trainees are encouraged to attend to their own emotional experience as learners and as clients. Essential areas of knowledge include general experiential therapy theory, emotion theory, the function of specific emotions, sources of emotional disorder, and cognitive–affective generating conditions for disorder, as outlined earlier in this book. Another important area of training concerns concepts pertinent to the therapeutic relationship. The development of perceptual skills involves learning to recognize the theoretical concepts as they appear in therapy, for the purpose of appropriate intervention.

Perceptual skills, such as recognition of process-diagnostic markers or attunement to the subtleties of vocal quality, are taught largely through observation of expert and peer videotapes of therapy (cf. Greenberg, 1990), as well as by learning certain research-based process-coding systems. Intervention skills are modelled by the trainer and acquired through supervised practice with peers and clinical work with volunteer "practice" clients. In the peer skills practice it is essential that trainees take the role of client in order to directly experience the impact of various interventions. This enhances their awareness of their own functioning and is an important aspect of developing empathic understanding of client processes.

As much as possible, the training process models the process of EFT intervention itself. First safety is established, and this is followed by an integration of conceptual and experiential learning. Early stages of training are also a good time to focus on issues of avoidance and interruption of experience, because these are naturally occurring phenomena for trainees at that time.

Trainees learn to work with different emotions by focusing on their own subjective experience of emotion. They are directed to attend to their own bodily experience, wants and needs, beliefs, memories, images, reactions of self and others, and specific situational triggers associated with particular emotional experiences. This is the focus of practice therapy sessions when the trainee is taking the role of client or in group discussions. Students also discuss their previous struggles and successes, as therapists in different clinical situations, working with clients' emotions. This provides a broad context for exploring the relevance of emotion in therapy process and therapeutic change.

One major goal of training in EFT is to help students become aware of and comfortable with their own emotional experience. This is essential before they can be aware of and comfortable with the emotional experience of others. In addition, trainees are encouraged to explore their strengths, weaknesses, and interpersonal styles and how these effect their work as therapists. For example, some find it difficult to intensify anger, whereas others find approaching and responding to emotional pain or sadness more challenging. Some are patient and reserved and need to learn to be more active; others are rather dominant and assertive and need to learn to be more responsive. We ask students to identify their strengths and weaknesses and their learning goals at the beginning of the training program. These are reference points for ongoing feedback.

Relationship Issues

Training programs usually have at least one module that is devoted to relationship issues. This includes observing videotapes of resolving relational issues such as ruptures, misunderstandings, and client reluctance to engage in active interventions. One issue that frequently arises in training is knowing when to encourage or momentarily abandon the use of active interventions. Although trainees usually do not have opportunities to practice these skills until they are working with real clients, they need to be aware that these issues inevitably will arise and of EFT's client-centered and collaborative approach to dealing with them.

The use of therapeutic touch is another issue that often is a topic for discussion in training groups. In working with emotion, touching a client's hand or shoulder, for example, can be helpful in relaxing tension and in supporting a person through grief and pain. However, knowledge of issues related to the ethics of touch as well as awareness of clients' possible fears and responses to touch requires clinical training. Four factors associated with clients' positive and negative evaluations of touch in psychotherapy have been identified (Horton, Clance, Sterk-Elifson, & Emshoff, 1995): (1) clarity regarding boundaries; (2) congruence of touch; (3) the client's perception of being in control of physical contact; and (4) the client's perception that touch is for his or her benefit rather than the therapist's. Clinicians in practice need to inquire whether the client would like to be touched at a particular moment. This should be done nonintrusively and quickly, without deflecting the process or creating an issue. Feedback from clients in posttherapy interviews has indicated that touch can be a powerful new experience for clients. However, touch is a complex subject that will not be discussed further here except to say that, at times, touch can be helpful and withholding touch can be harmful. Trainees need an opportunity to discuss the practical, ethical, and legal issues and their own feelings and concerns regarding therapeutic touch.

Intervention Skills

Training in EFT involves learning a fundamental empathic way of being as well as learning specific responding skills. An empathic way of being involves developing attitudes of empathy, unconditional positive regard, and genuineness (Rogers, 1957). Training and supervision in addition focus on intentional intervention, that is, conceptual understanding of dysfunctional processes and mechanisms of change, and how a particular intervention or therapist operation will bring about the desired process of change. Although we have studied particular types of interventions such as empty-chair work, EFT is not aligned with particular techniques except as they are vehicles for bringing about effective client processes. Training and supervision focuses on both intentions and the implementation of skills, fine-tuning perceptual and responding skills and technique, with attention to specificity and detail.

Many students enter training programs with the common view that empathic responses are simply supportive or maintenance responses, forming the background for the "real" or intense work of therapy. This can be especially true for trainees who are particularly attracted to the active interventions used in EFT. Basic texts on counseling and therapy skills reinforce this view by citing examples of empathic responses that often are clichéd, oversimplified, and trivial. For example, in an official preparatory course for an A.P.A. state Psychology Licensure Examination, an illustration of empathic responding in the section on client-centered therapy was as follows: "When a client says, 'I hate my father,' the therapist says, 'You feel that you hate him?' " In our experience, one of the most difficult tasks for trainees in EFT is to learn to move beyond this simplistic and sterile type of empathic reflection (cf. Bohart & Greenberg, 1997; Greenberg & Elliott, 1997). Trainees consistently remark that they had no idea of the complexity and subtlety of empathic responding. They come to appreciate and use empathic responding as a complex and sophisticated means of intervention designed to help clients make sense of their experience, which is much more difficult than simply reflecting back or asking a client how he or she feels. Trainees learn to use empathic responding not only to establish rapport but as an active intervention for realizing many of the intervention principles—directing and redirecting attention to internal experience, symbolizing the meaning of experience, and intensifying and responding to intentions.

In addition to empathy, certain skills are taught that facilitate the successful implementation of active interventions (Greenberg & Kahn, 1978). Trainees, for example, when implementing empty-chair work, are instructed to take a nonintrusive seating position, somewhat back from clients' lines of vision, so clients can easily ignore the therapist when they focus on the other chair. To promote the chair dialogues, therapists also need to learn to only minimally engage in interactive responding, and rather to give ongoing process directives that guide the client to engage in the task—for example, when speaking to her or his imagined father in the empty chair, "tell him how much you needed his support." This requires being exquisitely attuned to the client's internal processes so that directives are in synchrony with client experience and keep the process flowing rather than disrupting it with inaccurate responses.

Successfully implementing the active interventions also requires trainee understanding of the importance and value of the active interventions, independent of the interaction with the therapist. In the case of empty-chair work, for example, contact with the imagined other serves an evocative function that deepens experiencing and brings the emotion scheme alive.

Following versus Leading

Training involves learning the dialectical balance between following and leading, between empathic listening and process directiveness, between focusing in the moment and a more global task focus, as well as learning how to maintain the balance between directing attention to internal experience and directing active expression. However, process directiveness, by definition, always is guided by attunement to the client's internal process moment by moment because directives are guided by the client's changing states.

SUPERVISION

Supervision with real clients is the final stage in learning to implement the principles of EFT. Supervision is oriented toward fine-tuning the therapist's conceptual, perceptual, and intervention skills. The focus on moment-by-moment client processes needs to be balanced with skills in problem conceptualization and formulation. It is essential to generate broad but flexible intervention plans for a particular client and discuss possible directions for the next session or phase of treatment. Supervision itself becomes less instructional and more discussion oriented as the therapist gains in experience.

In supervision of therapy with real clients, trainees are faced with complex relationship issues that do not arise in training programs. Supervisees learn how to handle sensitive relationship issues in a way that is consistent with EFT (Kiesler, 1982a, 1982b; Safran, Muran, & Sanistag, 1994), to assess and accommodate individual client needs for structure, control, or pacing. They are helped to deal empathically and with immediacy to alliance ruptures and misunderstandings, control issues, clients reluctance to engage in active interventions, and difficult interpersonal styles. In all cases, the overarching principles are unconditional positive regard, genuineness, immediacy, and collaboration. Relationship training involves learning how to collaborate with clients on the goals and tasks of therapy in order to establish a working alliance. Supervisees are encouraged to spend the first three or four sessions on relationship building, collaboratively reaching an understanding of underlying generating conditions for pain and bad feelings, and establishing goals for the therapy and realistic expectations for change.

Supervisees are encouraged to specify, in concrete terms, their understanding of the client's problem or processing difficulties, the affective task that needs to be accomplished, how EFT and particular interventions can help, what is the next step in resolving the task, and what resolution will mean for this particular client.

CONCLUSION

Training and supervision in EFT provides trainees with encouragement and support, and builds on their existing strengths and knowledge base so they can successfully implement this model of therapy. Supervision has increased our confidence in this treatment approach—an essentially collaborative, person- and experience-centered approach that relies on the healthy and adaptive nature of human emotions. In this book we have sought to explicate, as specifically as possible, the theoretical framework underlying this emotionally focused approach to therapy, as well as to bring the theory alive through the use of clinical examples.

References

American Psychiatric Association. (1994). *Diagnostic and statistical manual of mental disorders* (4th ed.). Washington, DC: Author.

Barlow, D. H. (1985). The dimensions of anxiety disorders. In A. H. Tuma & J. D. Maser (Eds.), *Anxiety and the anxiety disorders.* Hillsdale, NJ: Erlbaum.

Barnard, P. J., & Teasdale, J. D. (1991). Interacting cognitive subsystems: A systematic approach to cognitive–affective interaction and change. *Cognition and Emotion, 5*(1), 1–39.

Beck, A. T. (1976). *Cognitive therapy and the emotional disorders.* New York: International Universities Press.

Benjamin, L. S. (1993). Every psychopathology is a gift of love (Presidential Address at the Annual International Meeting of the Society for Psychotherapy Research). *Psychotherapy Research, 3*(1), 1–24.

Benjamin, L. S. (1996). *Interpersonal diagnosis and treatment of personality disorders* (2nd ed.). New York: Guilford Press.

Bergin, A., & Garfield, S. (Eds.). (1994). *Handbook of psychotherapy and behavior change* (4th ed.). New York: Wiley.

Bernet, M. (1995). *Styles in perception of affect scale.* Brooklyn, NY: The SIPOAS Project.

Blaney, P. H. (1986). Affect and memory: A review. *Psychological Bulletin, 99,* 229–246.

Blatt, S. J., & Maroudas, C. (1992). Convergence of psychoanalytic and cognitive behavioral theories of depression. *Psychoanalytic Psychology, 9,* 157–190.

Bohart, A., & Greenberg, L. S. (1997). *Empathy reconsidered: Developments in psychotherapy.* Washington, DC: American Psychological Association.

Bolger, L. (1996). *The subjective experience of transformation through pain in adult children of alcoholics.* Unpublished doctoral dissertation, York University, Toronto, Ontario, Canada.

Bordin, E. S. (1979). The generalizability of the psychoanalytic concept of the working alliance. *Psychotherapy: Theory, Research and Practice, 16,* 252–260.

Bowlby, J. (1988). *A secure base.* New York: Basic Books.

Charney, D. S., Deutsch, A. Y., Krystal, J. H., Southwick, S. M., & David, M. (1993). Psychology mechanisms of posttraumatic stress disorder. *Archives of General Psychiatry, 50*(4), 294–305.

Clark, D. M., & Teasdale, J. D. (1982). Diurnal variation in clinical depression and accessibility of memories of positive and negative experiences. *Journal of Abnormal Psychology, 91*(2), 87–95.

Dalrup, R. J., Beutler, L. E., Engle, D., & Greenberg, L. S. (1988). *Focused expressive psychotherapy: Freeing the overcontrolled patient.* New York: Guilford Press.

Damasio, A. (1994). *Descartes' error: Emotion, reason, and the human brain.* New York: Putnam.

Darwin, C. (1955). *The expression of emotions in man and animal.* New York: Philosophical Library. (Original work published 1872)

Ekman, P., & Davidson, R. J. (1994). *The nature of emotion: Fundamental questions.* New York: Oxford University Press.

Ekman, P., & Friesen, W. V. (1975). *Unmasking the face.* Englewood Cliffs, NJ: Prentice-Hall.

Elliott, R., Flipovich, H., Harrigan, L., Gaynor, J., Reimschuessel, C., & Zapadka, J. K. (1982). Measuring response empath: The development of a multi-component rating scale. *Journal of Counseling Psychology, 29,* 379–387.

Ellis, A. (1962). *Reason and emotion in psychotherapy.* New York: Lyle Stewart.

Foa, E. B., & Kozak, M. J. (1986). Emotional processing of fear: Exposure of corrective information. *Psychological Bulletin, 99,* 20–35.

Frank, J. D. (1963). *Persuasion and healing: A comparative study of psychotherapy.* Baltimore: Johns Hopkins University Press.

Freud, S. (1963). The unconscious. *Standard Edition, 14,* 159–215. (Original work published 1915)

Frijda, N. H. (1986). *The emotions.* Cambridge, England: Cambridge University Press.

Gendlin, E. T. (1962). *Experiencing and the creation of meaning.* New York: Free Press of Glencoe.

Gendlin, E. T. (1964). A theory of personality change. In P. Worchel & D. Byrne (Eds.), *Personality change.* New York: Wiley.

Gendlin, E. T. (1974). Client-centered and experiential psychotherapy. In D. A. Wexler & L. N. Rice (Eds.), *Innovations in client-centered therapy*. New York: Wiley.

Gendlin, E. T. (1981). *Focusing*. New York: Bantam Books.

Gendlin, E. T. (1996). *A focusing approach to psychotherapy*. New York: Guilford Press.

Goldman, R. (1995, June). *The relationship between depth of experiencing and outcome in a depressed population*. Paper presented at the meeting of the Society for Psychotherapy Research, Vancouver, British Columbia, Canada.

Goldman, R., & Greenberg, L. S. (1992). Comparison of an integrated systemic and emotionally focused approach to couples therapy. *Journal of Consulting and Clinical Psychology, 60*, 962–969.

Goldman, R., & Greenberg, L. S. (1995). Case formulation. *In Session: Psychotherapy in Practice, 1*(2), 35–51.

Goldman, R., & Greenberg, L. S. (1997). Case formulation in Process Experiential Therapy. In T. D. Eells (Ed.), *Handbook of psychotherapy case formulation*. New York: Guilford Press.

Goldstein, K. (1939). *The organism*. The Hague: Nijhoff.

Goldstein, K. (1951). On emotions: Considerations from the organismic point of view. *Journal of Psychology, 221*, 226–227.

Gordon Walker, J., Johnson, S., Manion, I., & Cloutier, P. (1996). Emotionally focused marital interventions for couples with chronically ill children. *Journal of Consulting and Clinical Psychology, 64*, 1029–1036.

Greenberg, L. S. (1979). Resolving splits: The two-chair technique. *Psychotherapy: Theory, Research and Practice, 16*, 310–318.

Greenberg, L. S. (1984). A task-analysis of intrapersonal conflict resolution. In L. N. Rice & L. S. Greenberg (Eds.), *Patterns of change: Intensive analysis of psychotherapy process*. New York: Guilford Press.

Greenberg, L. S. (1990). *Integrative psychotherapy–Part v. An interview with Dr. Greenberg* [Film]. Corona del Mar, CA: Psychoeducational Films

Greenberg, L. S. (1991). Research on the process of change. *Psychotherapy Research, 1*, 14–24.

Greenberg, L. S. (1993). Emotion and change processes in psychotherapy. In M. Lewis & J. M. Haviland (Eds.), *Handbook of emotions*. New York: Guilford Press.

Greenberg, L. S. (1994). The investigation of change: Its measurement and explanation. In R. L. Russell (Ed.), *Reassessing psychotherapy research*. New York: Guilford Press.

Greenberg, L. S. (1995). The use of observational coding in family therapy research: Comment on Alexander et al. *Journal of Family Psychology, 9*(4), 366–370.

Greenberg, L. S., & Elliott, R. (1997). Varieties of empathic responding. In A. Bohart & L. S. Greenberg (Eds.), *Empathy reconsidered.* Washington, DC: American Psychological Association.

Greenberg, L. S., Elliott, R., & Foerster, F. S. (1991). Essential processes in the psychotherapeutic treatment of depression. In D. McCann & N. Endler (Eds.), *Depression: Developments in theory, research and practice* (pp. 157–185). Toronto: Thompson.

Greenberg, L. S., & Foerster, F. S. (1996). Resolving unfinished business: The process of change. *Journal of Consulting and Clinical Psychology, 64*(3), 439–446.

Greenberg, L., Ford, C., Alden, L., & Johnson, S. (1992). In session change processes in emotionally focused therapy for couples. *Journal of Consulting and Clinical Psychology, 60,* 1124–1132.

Greenberg, L. S., & Hirscheimer, K. (1994). *Relating degree of resolution of unfinished business to outcome.* Paper presented at the meeting of the North American Society for Psychotherapy Research, Santa Fe, NM.

Greenberg, L. S., & Johnson, S. M. (1988). *Emotionally focused therapy for couples.* New York: Guilford Press.

Greenberg, L. S., & Kahn, S. (1978). Experimentation: A Gestalt approach to counselling. *Canadian Counsellor, 13,* 23-27.

Greenberg, L. S., & Korman, L. (1993). Integrating emotion in psychotherapy integration. *Journal of Psychotherapy Integration, 3*(3), 249–265.

Greenberg, L. S., & Pascual-Leone, J. (1995). A dialectical constructivist approach to experiential change. In R. Neimeyer & M. Mahoney (Eds.), *Constructivism in psychotherapy.* Washington, DC: American Psychological Association.

Greenberg, L. S., & Pascual-Leone, J. (1997). *Emotion in the creation of personal meaning.* In M. Power & C. Bervin (Eds.), Transformation of meaning. Chichester: Wiley.

Greenberg, L. S., Rice, L. N., & Elliott, R. (1993). *Facilitating emotional change: The moment-by-moment process.* New York: Guilford Press.

Greenberg, L. S., & Safran, J. D. (1981). Encoding and cognitive therapy: Changing what clients attend to. *Psychotherapy: Theory, Research and Practice, 8,* 163-169.

Greenberg, L., & Safran, J. D. (1984a). Integrating affect and cognition: A perspective on the process of therapeutic change. *Cognitive Therapy and Research, 8,* 559–578.

Greenberg, L. S., & Safran, J. D. (1984b). Hot cognition: Emotion coming in from the cold. A reply to Rachman and Mahoney. *Cognitive Therapy and Research, 8,* 591–598.

Greenberg, L. S., & Safran, J. D. (1987). *Emotion in psychotherapy: Affect, cognition, and the process of change.* New York: Guilford Press.

Greenberg, L. S., & Safran, J. D. (1989). Emotion in psychotherapy. *American Psychologist, 44,* 19–29.

Greenberg, L. S., & Watson, J. (in press). Client-centered and process experiential treatment of depression: A preliminary comparative outcome study. *Psychotherapy Research.*

Greenberg, L. S., & Webster, M. (1982). Resolving decisional conflict by means of two-chair dialogue and empathic reflection at a split in counseling. *Journal of Counseling Psychology, 29,* 478–477.

Guidano, V. F. (1987). *Complexity of the self: A developmental approach to psychopathology and therapy.* New York: Guilford Press.

Guidano, V. F. (1991a). *The self in process: Toward a post-rationalist cognitive therapy.* New York: Guilford Press.

Guidano, V. F. (1991b). Affective change events in a cognitive therapy system approach. In J. D. Safran & L. S. Greenberg (Eds.), *Emotion, psychotherapy, and change.* New York: Guilford Press.

Guidano, V. F. (1995). The constructivist psychotherapy: A theoretical framework. In R. Neimeyer & M. Mahoney (Eds.), *Constructivism in psychotherapy.* Washington, DC: American Psychological Association Press.

Herman, J. L. (1992). *Trauma and recovery.* New York: Basic Books.

Hillman, J. (1960). *Emotion: A comprehensive phenomenology of theories and their meanings for therapy.* Evanston, IL: Northwestern University Press.

Horowitz, M. (1986). *Stress response syndrome.* Northvale, NJ: Aronson.

Horton, J. A., Clance, P. R., Sterk-Elifson, C., & Enshoff, J. (1995). Touch in psychotherapy: A survey of patient's experiences. *Psychotherapy, 32*(3), 443–457.

Horvath, A. O., & Greenberg, L. S. (1994). *The working alliance: Theory, research and practice.* New York: Wiley.

Isen, A. (1984). Toward understanding the role of affect on cognition. In R. S. Wyer, Jr. & T. S. Krull (Eds.), *Handbook of social cognition* (Vol. 3). Hillsdale, NJ: Erlbaum.

Izard, C. E. (1979). *Emotion in personality and psychopathology,* New York: Plenum Press.

Izard, C. E. (1990). Personality, emotion expressions, and rapport. *Psychological Inquiry, 1*(4), 315–317.

Izard, C. E. (1991). *The psychology of emotions.* New York: Plenum Press.

Izard, C. E. (1993). Four systems for emotion activation: Cognitive and noncognitive processes. *Psychological Review, 100*(1), 68–90.

James, W. (1950). *The principles of psychology.* New York: Dover. (Original work published 1890)

Janoff-Bulman, R. (1992). *Shattered assumptions: Towards a new psychology of trauma.* New York: Free Press.

Jaspers, K. (1963). *General psychopathology* (J. Hoenig & M. W. Hamilton, Trans.). Chicago: University of Chicago Press.

Johnson, S. M., & Greenberg, L. S. (1985). Differential effects of experiential and problem solving interventions in resolving marital conflict. *Journal of Consulting and Clinical Psychology, 53,* 175–184.

Johnson, S., & Greenberg, G. L. (1988). Relating process to outcome in marital therapy. *Journal of Marital and Family Therapy, 14,* 175–183.

Kaufman, G. (1989). *The psychology of shame: Theory and treatment of shame-based syndromes.* New York: Springer.

Kiesler, D. J. (1982a). Interpersonal theory for personality and psychotherapy. In J. C. Anchin & D. J. Kiesler (Eds.), *Handbook of interpersonal psychotherapy.* Elmsford, NY: Pergamon Press.

Kiesler, D. J. (1982b). Confronting the client–therapist relationship in psychotherapy. In J. C. Anchin & D. J. Kiesler (Eds.), *Handbook of interpersonal psychotherapy.* Elmsford, NY: Pergamon Press.

Klein, M., Mathieu, P., Kiesler, D., & Gendlin, E. (1969). *The Experiencing Scale.* Madison, WI: Wisconsin Psychiatric Institute.

Kopp, C. B. (1989). Regulation of distress and negative emotions: A developmental view. *Developmental Psychology, 25*(3), 343–354.

Korman, L., & Greenberg, L. S. (1996). *Do emotions change in therapy? Measuring emotion episodes across treatment.* Paper presented at the meeting of the International Society for Research in Emotion, Toronto, Ontario, Canada.

Lazarus, R. S. (1986). Sensory systems and emotion: A model of affective processing: Comment. *Integrative Psychiatry, 4*(4), 245–247.

LeDoux, J. E. (1993). Emotional networks in the brain. In M. Lewis & J. M. Haviland (Eds.), *Handbook of emotions.* New York: Guilford Press.

LeDoux, J. E. (1994). Emotion, memory and the brain. *Scientific American, 27*(6), 32–39.

Leventhal, H. (1982). The integration of emotion and cognition: A view from the perceptual motor theory of emotion. In M. S. Clarke & S. T. Fiske (Eds.), *Affect and cognition: The 17th Annual Carnegie Symposium on Cognition.* Hillsdale, NJ: Erlbaum.

Leventhal, H. (1984). A perceptual-motor theory of emotion. In L. Berkowitz (Ed.), *Advances in experimental social psychology.* New York: Academic Press.

Lewin, K. (1935). *A dynamic theory of personality.* New York: McGraw-Hill.

Monsen, J. (1994). *Personality disorders and intensive psychotherapy focusing on affect-consciousness: A prospective follow-up study.* Monograph, University of Oslo, Blindern, Norway.

Nason, J. D. (1985). The psychotherapy of rage: Clinical and developmental perspectives. *Contemporary Psychoanalysis, 21*(2), 167–192.

Norcross, J. C., & Goldfried, M. R. (1992). *Handbook of psychotherapy integration.* New York: Basic Books.

Oatley, K. (1992). *Best land schemes: The psychotherapy of emotions.* New York: Cambridge University Press.

Oatley, K., & Jenkins, J. M. (1992). Human emotions: Function and dysfunction. *Annual Review of Psychology, 43,* 55–85.

Paivio, S. C. (1995). *Resolving unfinished business stemming from childhood abuse.* Paper presented at the meeting of the Society for Psychotherapy Research, Vancouver, British Columbia, Canada.

Paivio, S. C., & Greenberg, L. S. (1995). Resolving unfinished business: Experiential therapy using empty-chair dialogue. *Journal of Consulting and Clinical Psychology, 63*(3), 419–425.

Paivio, S. C., & Greenberg, L. S. (1997). Experintial theory of anxiety and depression. In W. F. Flack & J. D. Laird (Eds.), *Emotion in psychopathology: Theory and research.* New York: Oxford University Press.

Paivio, S. C., Lake, R. P., Nieuwenhuis, J. A., & Baskerville, S. (1996). *Emotional change processes in experiential therapy for the effects of childhood abuse.* Paper presented at the meeting of the Society for the Exploration of Psychotherapy Integration, Berkeley, CA.

Pascual-Leone, J. (1990a). An essay on wisdom: Toward organismic processes that make it possible. In R. J. Sternberg (Ed.), *Wisdom: Its nature, origins and development.* New York: Cambridge University Press.

Pascual-Leone, J. (1990b). Reflections on life-span intelligence, consciousness and ego development. In C. N. Alexander & E. Langer (Eds.), *Higher stages of human development.* New York: Oxford University Press.

Pascual-Leone, J. (1991). Emotions, development and psychotherapy: A dialectical-constructivist perspective. In J. D. Safran & L. S. Greenberg (Eds.), *Emotion, psychotherapy, and change.* New York: Guilford Press.

Pascual-Leone, J. (1992). The dynamic system reasoning: Comment. *Human Development, 35*(3), 138–141.

Pennebaker, J. W. (1989). Confession, inhibition and disease. In L. Berkowitz (Ed.), *Advances in experimental social psychology* (Vol. 22). New York: Academic Press.

Pennebaker, J. W. (1990). *Opening up: The healing power of confiding in others.* New York: Morrow.

Perls, F. S. (1969). *Gestalt therapy verbatim.* Lafayette, CA: Real People Press.

Perls, F. S. (1973). *The Gestalt approach and eyewitness to therapy.* Palo Alto, CA: Science and Behavior Books.

Perls, F. S., Hefferline, R., & Goodman, P. (1951). *Gestalt therapy.* New York: Dell.

Rice, L. N. (1974). *The evocative function of the therapist.* In L. N. Rice & D. A. Wexler (Eds.), *Innovations in client-centered therapy.* New York: Wiley.

Rice, L. N. (1984). Client tasks in client-centered therapy. In R. F. Levant & J. M. Shlien (Eds.), *Client-centered therapy and the person-centered approach: New directions in theory, research, and practice.* New York: Praeger.

Rogers, C. R. (1957). The necessary and sufficient condition of therapeutic personality change. *Journal of Consulting Psychology, 21,* 95–103.

Rogers, C. R. (1959). A theory of therapy, personality, and interpersonal relationships as developed in the client-centered framework. In S. Koch (Ed.), *Psychology: The study of a science* (Vol. 3). New York: McGraw-Hill.

Rossman, B. R. (1992). School-age children's perceptions of coping with distress: Strategies for emotion regulation and the moderation of adjustment. *Journal of Child Psychology and Psychiatry and Allied Disciplines, 33*(8), 1373–1397.

Safran, J. D., & Greenberg, L. S. (Eds.). (1991). *Emotion, psychotherapy, and change.* New York: Guilford Press.

Safran, J., Muran, C., & Sanistag., L. (1994). Resolving therapeutic alliance ruptures: A task analytic investigation. In A. Horvath & L. Greenberg (Eds.), *The working alliance: Theory, Research, and Practice.* New York: Wiley–Interscience.

Salovey, P., Hsee, C., & Mayer, J. D. (1993). Emotional intelligence and the self-regulation of affect. In D. M. Wegner & J. W. Pennebaker (Eds.), *Handbook of mental control.* Englewood Cliffs, NJ: Prentice-Hall.

Salovey, P., & Mayer, J. D. (1989). Emotional intelligence. *Imagination, Cognition and Personality, 9*(3), 185–211.

Sartre, J.-P. (1948). *The emotions: Outlines of a theory.* New York: Philosophical Library.

Scherer, K. R. (1984). On the nature and function of emotion: A component process approach. In K. R. Scherer & P. Ekman (Eds.), *Approaches to emotion.* Hillsdale, NJ: Erlbaum.

Simons, A. D., Garfield, S. L., & Murphy, G. E. (1984). The process of change in cognitive therapy and pharmacotherapy for depression: Changes in mood and cognition. *Archives of General Psychiatry, 41,* 45–51.

Smith, T. (1996, August). *Emotion diaries and depression.* Paper presented at the meeting of the International Society for Research in Emotion, Toronto, Ontario, Canada.

Sroufe, L. A. (1996). *Emotional development: The organization of emotional life in the early years.* New York: Cambridge University Press.

Stern, D. N. (1985). *The interpersonal world of the infant: A view from psychoanalysis and developmental psychology.* New York: Basic Books.

Teasdale, J. D., & Barnard, P. J. (1993). *Affect, cognition and change: Re-modelling depressive thought.* Trowbridge, England: Redwood Books.

Thompson, R. A. (1988). Emotion and self-regulation. In R. A. Thompson (Ed.), *Nebraska Symposium on Motivation: Vol. 36. Socioemotional development: Current theory and research in motivation.* Lincoln: University of Nebraska Press.

Tomkins, S. (1962). *Affect, imagery, and consciousness.* New York: Springer.

Tomkins, S. (1991). *Affect, imagery, and consciousness: Vol. 3. The negative affects: Anger and fear.* New York: Springer.

van der Kolk, B. (1996). The body keeps the score: Approaches to the psychobiology of posttraumatic stress disorder. In B. A. van der Kolk, A. C. McFarlane, & L. Weisaeth (Eds.), *Traumatic stress: The effects of overwhelming experience on mind, body, and society.* New York: Guilford Press.

Watson, J. C., & Greenberg, L. S. (1994). The alliance in experiential therapy: Enacting the relationship conditions. In A. O. Horvath & L. S. Greenberg (Eds.), *The working alliance: Theory, research and practice.* New York: Wiley.

Watson, J. C., & Greenberg, L. S. (1995). Emotion and cognition in experiential therapy: A dialectical–constructivist position. In H. Rosen & K. Kuhelwein (Eds.), *Constructing realities: Meaning making perspectives for psychotherapists.* New York: Jossey-Bass.

Watson, J. C., & Greenberg, L. S. (1996). Pathways to change in the psychotherapy of depression: Relating process to session change and outcome. *Psychotherapy, 33,* 262–274.

Watson, J. C., & Rennie, D. (1994). Qualitative analysis of client's subjective experience of significant moments during the explo-

ration of problematic reactions. *Journal of Counseling Psychology,*
41, 500–509.

Weiss, J., Sampson, H., & the Mount Zion Psychotherapy Research
Group. (1986). *The psychoanalytic process: Theory, clinical observa-*
tions, and empirical research. New York: Guilford Press.

Winnicott, D. W. (1965). *The maturational process and the facilitating*
environment. New York: International Universities Press.

Yontef, G. M., & Simkin, J. S. (1989). Gestalt therapy. In R. J. Corsini
& D. Wedding (Eds.), *Current psychotherapies.* Itasca, IL: Peacock.

Zajonc, R. B. (1980). Feeling and thinking: Preferences need no
inferences. *American Psychologist, 35,* 151–175.

Index